# Anxiety and Related Disorders Interview Schedule for DSM-5, Child and Parent Versions

# Anxiety and Related Disorders Interview Schedule for DSM-5, Child and Parent Versions

## Clinician Manual

Wendy K. Silverman
Anne Marie Albano

## with a supplement on Autism Spectrum Addendum

Connor M. Kerns
Wendy K. Silverman
Anne Marie Albano

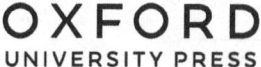

# OXFORD
## UNIVERSITY PRESS

Oxford University Press is a department of the University of Oxford. It furthers the University's objective of excellence in research, scholarship, and education by publishing worldwide. Oxford is a registered trade mark of Oxford University Press in the UK and certain other countries.

Published in the United States of America by Oxford University Press
198 Madison Avenue, New York, NY 10016, United States of America.

Library of Congress Cataloging-in-Publication Data
Names: Silverman, Wendy K., editor. | Albano, Anne Marie, editor.
Title: Anxiety and related disorders interview schedule for DSM-5, child and parent versions : clinician manual / Wendy K. Silverman, Anne Marie Albano.
Description: New York, NY : Oxford University Press, [2024] |
Series: Treatments that work | Includes bibliographical references and index.
Identifiers: LCCN 2021037328 (print) | LCCN 2021037329 (ebook) |
ISBN 9780199348343 (paperback) | ISBN 9780197585894 (epub) |
ISBN 9780197626160
Subjects: LCSH: Anxiety—Diagnosis—Handbooks, manuals, etc. |
Mental illness—Classification—Handbooks, manuals, etc. |
Interviewing in psychiatry.
Classification: LCC RC531 .B763 2023 (print) | LCC RC531 (ebook) |
DDC 616.85/22—dc23
LC record available at https://lccn.loc.gov/2021037328
LC ebook record available at https://lccn.loc.gov/2021037329

DOI: 10.1093/med-psych/9780199348343.001.0001

Printed by Integrated Books International, United States of America

# CONTENTS

# ABOUT THE ADIS DEVELOPERS

**Wendy K. Silverman** is the Alfred A. Messer Professor of Child Psychiatry, Professor of Psychology, and Director of the Yale Child Study Center Anxiety and Mood Disorders Program at Yale University School of Medicine. Dr. Silverman has published many scientific articles and book chapters, and five books. For the past three decades she has served as Principal Investigator of National Institute of Mental Health (NIMH) research grants to develop and evaluate novel treatments for childhood, a co-investigator on many other projects, and recipient of a NIMH mid-career development award (2005–2010) to support her research and her mentoring of trainees. Dr. Silverman served as Associate Editor and Editor of *Journal of Clinical Child and Adolescent Psychology*, Associate Editor of *Journal of Consulting and Clinical Psychology*, Co-Editor of *Clinical Psychology Review*, and Chairperson of an NIMH grant review panel. She is past president of the Society for Clinical Child and Adolescent Psychology of the American Psychological Association and is Board Certified in Clinical Child and Adolescent Psychology.

*Anne Marie Albano* is the Columbia University Clinic for Anxiety and Related Disorders Professor of Medical Psychology in Psychiatry at Columbia University Vagelos College of Physicians and Surgeons. She is Founder of the Columbia University Clinic for Anxiety and Related Disorders and Clinical Site Director of New York Presbyterian Hospital's Youth Anxiety Center. Dr. Albano is a Fellow of the American Psychological Association and the Association for Behavioral and Cognitive Therapies (ABCT), is a Founding Fellow of the Academy of Cognitive Therapy, and is Board Certified in Clinical Child and Adolescent Psychology. Dr. Albano served as a Principal Investigator of the National Institute of Mental Health (NIMH)-sponsored "Child/Adolescent Anxiety Multimodal Treatment Study" (CAMS) and the "Treatments for Adolescents with Depression Study" (TADS) randomized controlled clinical trials. In 2017 Dr. Albano was granted a Herbert O. Pardes M.D. Faculty Fellowship Award to support her treatment development research focused on emerging adults with anxiety. She received the 2015 ABCT Award for Outstanding Contributions by an Individual for Clinical Activities. Dr. Albano is a past president of the Society for Clinical Child and Adolescent Psychology of the American Psychological Association and past president of the Association for Behavioral and Cognitive Therapies (ABCT), past editor of *Cognitive and Behavioral Practice*, founding and past editor of *Evidence-Based Practice in Child and Adolescent Mental Health*, and past associate editor of the *Journal of Consulting and Clinical Psychology*. She has published many empirical articles and chapters and is the co-author of several cognitive behavioral treatment manuals published by Oxford University Press. ABCT offers an annual award established in Dr. Albano's name by a family to encourage the proliferation of evidence-based treatment, the Anne Marie Albano Early Career Award for Excellence in the Integration of Science and Practice.

Together, Drs. Albano and Silverman devoted their careers to understanding and treating anxiety in children, adolescents, and young adults. Their decades of direct clinical work with youth and families, coupled with their research endeavors and training of an extensive cadre of clinicians and clinical scientists, are emblematic of their shared goal to advance the understanding and treatment of anxiety and its disorders in children, adolescents, and young adults.

# CONTRIBUTOR

*Connor M. Kerns*, is an Associate Professor and Director of the Anxiety Stress and Autism Program (ASAP) in the Department of Psychology at the University of British Columbia. Dr. Kerns's clinical practice and research are focused on the assessment and treatment of anxiety and stress-related disorders in children on the autism spectrum. She has published extensively on these topics, including numerous articles and chapters and an edited book, *Anxiety in Children and Adolescents with Autism Spectrum Disorder: Evidence-Based Assessment and Treatment*. Dr. Kerns is a Killam Research Fellow and the recipient of early career awards from the National Institute of Child and Human Development (NICHD) and Michael Smith Foundation for Health Research. She has also received funding (as principal or co-investigator) from the National Institute of Mental Health, Canadian Institute for Health Research, Autism Science Foundation, Social Sciences and Humanities Research Council, and Canadian Foundation of Innovation to support her research.

# CHAPTER 1

## ANXIETY AND RELATED DISORDERS INTERVIEW SCHEDULE FOR DSM-5, CHILD AND PARENT VERSIONS

*Wendy K. Silverman and Anne Marie Albano*

## INTRODUCTION

The Anxiety and Related Disorders Interview Schedule for DSM-5 (ADIS-5), Child and Parent Versions, was updated for use in clinical practice and in research trials to provide for the differential diagnosis of the full range of psychiatric and behavioral health disorders in children and adolescents (hereafter referred to as "children") while also establishing the child's full psychiatric history. This version, as in the original ADIS interviews,[1,2] is based on the fifth edition of the American Psychiatric Association's *Diagnostic and Statistical Manual of Mental Disorders* (DSM-5),[3] allowing the clinician to rule out alternative diagnoses and establish the child's present record of psychiatric disorder. The ADIS provides quantifiable data concerning the symptoms, severity, etiology, and course of disorders. These data can be useful for case conceptualization; for pre-, mid-, or post-treatment evaluations for tracking clinical course and response; and for research purposes.

## ADAPTATIONS OF THE ADIS FOR DSM-5

The ADIS-5 provides for both present and, in the Parent Version, lifetime diagnoses. A full range of disorders is included in the ADIS-5, including diagnostic categories that were introduced in the DSM-5.

The Parent Version also contains a module to gather information about the child's development, functioning, and previous clinical and educational evaluations/services received by the child. This information, in conjunction with information obtained from the diagnostic sections of the ADIS, allows the clinician to complete the Developmental and Clinical Timeline (see Figures 1.1 and 1.2 on pp. 39–40 of this Clinician Manual). The timeline is provided to track the onset of key symptoms and diagnoses, achievement of developmental milestones, educational

[1] Silverman, W. K., & Nelles, W. B. (1988). The Anxiety Disorders Interview Schedule for Children. *Journal of the American Academy of Child and Adolescent Psychiatry, 27,* 772–778.

[2] Silverman, W. K., & Albano, A. M. (1996). *The Anxiety Disorders Interview Schedule for DSM-IV, Child and Parent Versions.* Oxford University Press.

[3] American Psychiatric Association. (2013). *Diagnostic and statistical manual of mental disorders* (5th edition). APA Press.

and therapeutic intervention and supports, and life events. The timeline also allows the clinician to organize clinical information and view a summary of the child's symptoms and functioning to inform the case formulation and treatment plan.

Even if a child does not meet minimum criteria for diagnosis(es) at the present time, the ADIS Parent Version allows the interviewer to skip to a lifetime inquiry section designed to ask whether there has ever been a time when the child evidenced the disorder. In addition, age of onset of the various disorders is ascertained. This clinical information about onset and previous episodes allows for the tracking of patterns of onset and remission, comorbidity, and course of the disorders to the present time.

Also new to the ADIS Parent Version for DSM-5 is a separate supplement for the assessment of the unique symptom presentation of anxiety in youth on the autism spectrum and developmental disorders adapted by Connor Kerns. See Chapter 2, "Anxiety and Related Disorders Interview Schedule for Parent Version: Autism Spectrum Addendum (ADIS/ASA)," starting on p. x of this Clinician Manual.

## ADIS DIAGNOSTIC PROCEDURES

The ADIS for DSM-5 follows the same procedures established for the original ADIS-C interview. The evaluator conducts separate interviews with the child and the parent(s). The interviews may be conducted in random order (either parent or child first) by the same evaluator. It is important to refrain from using any information gained from one informant to influence the response of the second informant. Diagnoses are derived separately for the child interview and parent interview, based on the information gained from the respective informant and the interviewer's knowledge of DSM diagnoses. Guidelines are provided for combining the child and parent information into summary diagnosis(es) known as the Composite Diagnosis (see pp. 7–12 in this Clinician Manual). The Composite Diagnosis forms the "working" diagnosis to guide treatment planning or study entry, if the ADIS is used in research.

### Semi-Structured Format

All information or questions to be directed to the child and parents are printed in **boldfaced type**. These questions can be repeated verbatim but allow the interviewer to use clinical judgment to adapt questions to maximize informant cooperation as well as reliable and accurate reporting. Also, for each question, take into account informant age; developmental level; and cultural, ethnic/race, and gender identification in a sensitive and effective manner. As necessary, the interviewer may probe further or reword or rephrase a question. Also, if in doubt, do not skip a section.

The relationship of the adult informant to the child informant also is helpful to consider. For example, a noncustodial caretaker (e.g., guardian, foster parent) may have limited information about the child's functioning in certain contexts and over time due to reduced firsthand observations. Under these circumstances, the interviewer might note when the response is limited or questionable and for what reason.

## Use of the ADIS with Non–English-Speaking Informants

Real-time translation of any ADIS section or question for use with non–English-speaking informants is not recommended. The acquisition of accurate information is largely dependent on language usage in particular cultural and colloquial contexts. American English terminology and structure also do not translate directly to other languages and cultures. Concepts, especially mental health concepts such as "panic attack," "depression," and "obsessions," have different meanings cross-culturally, in addition to there being specific manifestations of clinical symptoms unique to some cultural groups. Although a translator may be the only option in some cases, the information gained may not accurately reflect the intent of the question or the experience of the informant. Translation of the ADIS into languages other than American English requires approval by Oxford University Press in consultation with Drs. Albano and Silverman.

# STRUCTURE AND FORMAT OF THE ADIS

This section describes the various modules and features of the ADIS.

## Introduction

The ADIS begins with an introductory module for building a common language and understanding between the child and interviewer and for training the child on the use of the Feelings Thermometer, the visual prompt accompanying the ADIS to enhance accuracy of self-report. The Parent Version contains an abbreviated introductory section. The Feelings Thermometer also is often helpful to use with parents as a means for enhancing accuracy and consistency of report.

The child interview begins with a presentation and explanation of the Feelings Thermometer, showing the child how the thermometer increases in "degrees" from 0 (none, not at all) to 8 (very, very much). Verbal anchors accompany the even numbers on the thermometer. Children are asked to say aloud or to point to the thermometer to rate their level of fear, distress, and interference.

**Feelings Thermometer**

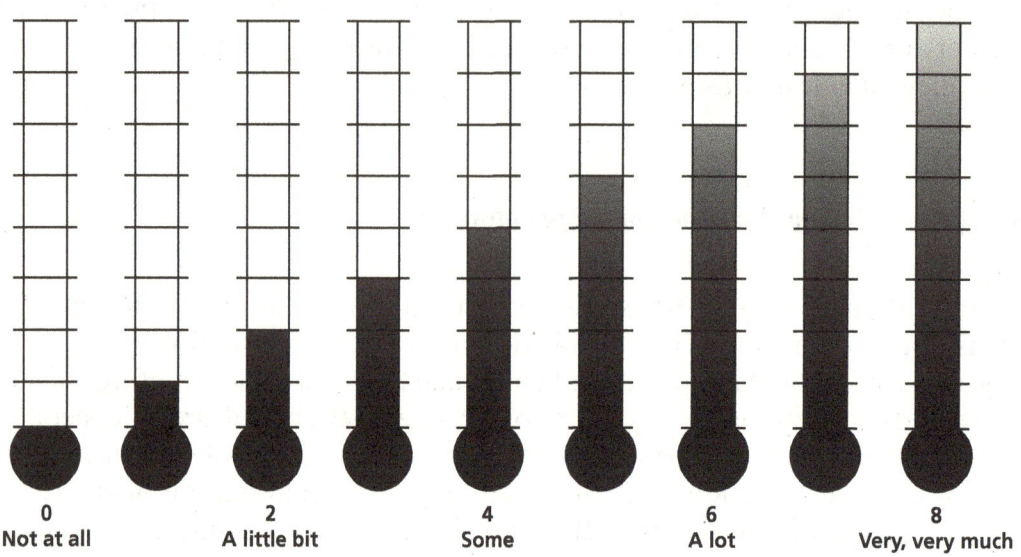

| 0 | | 2 | | 4 | | 6 | | 8 |
| Not at all | | A little bit | | Some | | A lot | | Very, very much |

---

## Clinician Note

*While administering the ADIS, interviewers should repeat aloud the child's, adolescent's, or parent's rating to ensure accuracy and to allow the rating to be heard on any recording being generated for clinical supervision or for assessment of study reliability and integrity.*

---

To practice using the Feelings Thermometer, we provide the child with examples that are not focused on the referring problem. Using the language/word most comfortable and age-appropriate for the child, ask:

1. *Not at all*: How anxious/nervous/scared would you feel (playing with your favorite toy; listening to music) at home or in your room?

2. *Some*: How upset would you feel if you misplaced your homework?

3. *A lot*: How anxious/nervous/scared would you feel watching a horror movie alone, at home, in the dark, during a storm?

4. *Very, very much*: How anxious/nervous/scared would you feel if you had to jump out of an airplane?

## School History and School Refusal Behavior

The first section of the Parent Interview is designed to obtain basic information about the child's school history and performance, followed by an assessment of school refusal behavior. The Child Interview is focused on the experience of anxiety and related feelings pertaining to school, and assesses patterns of school refusal. The interviewer follows a series of questions to evaluate whether school attendance is problematic for the child. Because the ADIS is a semi-structured interview, it is expected that the wording or phrasing of questions will be adapted by the clinician to meet the developmental level and/or cultural background of the child. *The School Refusal section is not a diagnostic section.*

### Clinician Note

*In the ADIS-5, the School Refusal section is shortened and does not include a list of situations/activities that may prompt anxiety and school avoidance. These situations are assessed as they occur in the context of the individual diagnostic modules.*

## Diagnostic Modules

The ADIS contains separate diagnostic modules for the DSM-5 disorders, beginning with the anxiety disorders. These modules are designed to orient the informant to the issue in question ("*Some children have trouble being away from their parents or home*") and provide prompts for the interviewer to skip to the next module if a minimum number of symptoms have not been endorsed. Interviewers need to use discretion when making use of the "skips;" for example, it might be appropriate to skip in some clinical settings but not when used for research purposes. In addition, as noted above, clinicians who wish to examine prior episodes of a condition or to develop a diagnostic timeline of prior symptoms may wish to continue while making note of the inquiry being framed in a past-history context.

The ADIS diagnostic modules are structured in the following format.

### *Initial Inquiry*

This section provides a summary statement of the disorder in question to familiarize the informant with the diagnostic category (e.g., separation anxiety, social anxiety, depression) and to move the informant away from previously discussed categories or other areas of inquiry. It is important to focus the child or parent on the construct in question so as to separate the different types of anxiety and other DSM conditions that may coexist but at different levels of intensity and interference.

### *Symptom Ratings*

The informant is asked to identify the presence of relevant symptoms and at times to provide ratings of the level of feeling (fear, anxiety, worry) associated with the symptom. In some sections, the informant is also asked to rate the degree of avoidance of certain situations or activities. For example, in Social Anxiety Disorder, the informant is asked to rate how much they avoid situations such as giving oral reports, joining conversations, or asking for help.

### Interference Ratings

Each diagnosis in the DSM-5 requires the presence of clinically significant distress or impairment in functioning. Upon gathering the information necessary to make the diagnosis (minimum number of symptoms and time period met), the informant is asked to provide a summary rating of the degree to which the problem leads to distress or interference in a broad range of functioning (self-care, school, peers, family). The informant may use the Feelings Thermometer to provide a global rating of the level of interference associated with the symptoms within each diagnostic category on a scale of 0 (not at all) to 8 (very, very much).

### Sequencing the Assessment of Symptoms on Multiple Dimensions

In diagnostic sections where the symptoms, severity ratings, and interference ratings are listed in columnar form (e.g., Social Anxiety Disorder, Panic Disorder, Specific Phobia, Generalized Anxiety Disorder [GAD]), the interviewer needs to inquire about the presence, severity, and degree of interference for symptoms in a coherent manner and facilitate the informant's understanding. That is, the interviewer may first inquire "down" the list to assess for presence of the symptom (yes or no) or fear/anxiety rating (0–8), and then return to the list to inquire about levels of distress or avoidance for each endorsed situation. Alternatively, the interviewer may first inquire "across" each symptom—such as when an informant endorses "yes" to an item, the interviewer may then inquire about fear, distress, and avoidance for that item—before moving down the list to the next situation. The decision to go "down" versus "across" the list is left to the interviewer and their judgment on how best a respondent understands the concepts and can work through the symptom lists. It is recommended that the clinician be consistent in going down or across in soliciting ratings, to avoid confusing the informant.

### Accuracy and Anomalies in Ratings

At times a respondent will report a rating that seems out of range in relation to the symptom report. A child who reports being nervous while giving oral reports but does not avoid school or the situation of presenting in front of the class, and rates their fear at a level of 7, is not using the range of the rating scale as intended. A fear rating of 7 is at the near extreme level and is typically accompanied by much avoidance and upset. Children may over-rate or under-rate fear for a variety of reasons related to their level of cognitive development, overall distress, intention to minimize or exaggerate, timing in relation to the most recent or distant fear or worry episode, and other factors. Clinicians are advised to consider these and other issues that impact self-report in youth and to address this in the clinical note as well as in assigning Confidence Ratings (see below) for the interview.

Also, a child who provides the same thermometer rating repeatedly for different symptoms and/or interference rating (i.e., "response sets") is also something for the interviewer to address. For example, if a child provides the same rating for each situation in the social anxiety section, the interviewer should ask, "*You rated giving an oral report as a 5 on the thermometer, and you also gave a 5 to joining in on a conversation, and a 5 for asking the teacher for help. Do these situations lead you to feel the same amount of (fear, anxiety)? Is one of these situations worse or easier for you than the others?*" The child may also be asked to rank order the situations and then assign a rating: "*How would you rank these situations from easiest to hardest? Now, what thermometer rating would you give to each?*"

Parents may also over-rate or under-rate their child's level of fear or anxiety. It is important to remind an adult respondent that their ratings of the child's fear or anxiety should be based on comparison to "other kids" of similar age to the child. For example, "*When you tell me that your child is very afraid of answering questions in class, is your child much more afraid than other kids of similar age?*" Some parents may not have experience with other youth and also may have different expectations or understanding of what is typical for a developmental age. It is important for the interviewer to ask questions to determine if there are limits or biases to the parents' knowledge in these areas.

## ASSIGNING DIAGNOSES, INTERFERENCE RATINGS, CONFIDENCE RATINGS, AND CLINICIAN SEVERITY RATINGS

Interference Ratings (IRs) are assigned for each diagnosis reflecting the degree of distress and interference reported by the child during the Child Interview and separately during the Parent Interview. These ratings are then combined into a Composite Diagnosis with associated severity ratings by the clinician.

The ADIS provides for separate diagnoses from the Child Interview and Parent Interview based on informants' symptom reports:

1. Symptom circles are checked if a symptom is present.

2. Criterion diamonds are checked if diagnostic criteria or symptom counts are met.

3. The Diagnosis star is then checked if all diagnostic criteria for a disorder are met.

At the end of each diagnostic module, the clinician asks for a rating of interference and distress. The Child Interference Rating (CIR) and Parent Interference Rating (PIR) will then be combined into the final Clinician Severity Rating (CSR) by the clinician.

The IR is a rating of symptom severity and disability as reported by the child or parent. At times, the CIR or PIR may not accurately reflect the level of disability that was reported during the diagnostic module. That is, a child or parent may under-estimate or over-estimate the degree of impairment. A Confidence Rating for each diagnosis is also assigned (see "Confidence Ratings" on p. x) to assist the clinician in refining the final Composite Diagnosis and overall level of impairment.

Following the completion of each interview, the interviewer will review each diagnostic section and note whether the minimum number of symptoms has been met and examine the associated IR offered by the informant. Based on the information gathered during the relevant section and on the *interviewer's* knowledge of normative levels of anxiety (or mood symptoms, variations in attention, etc.), in addition to levels of increasing severity and disability associated with the diagnosis, and considering the level of confidence in the reports and IRs, the interviewer then combines the information from the child and parent interviews for each diagnostic category endorsed by the informants.

## Caveats to the Process of Assigning IRs

In reviewing the obtained symptom report and the IRs, some respondents will provide a fairly accurate rating for interference, whereas others may under-report or over-report distress. For example, suppose a 10-year-old child endorses fears of being separated from parents, a fear that something bad will happen to the child if not with the parents, an inability to sleep alone, nightmares about separations, and an inability to visit the home of friends, among other symptoms that have been consistent and worsening over the past 2 years. The child in this case reports meeting more than the minimum number of symptoms and relevant time period. However, despite summarizing the endorsed symptoms for the child and asking them to think about using the whole range of the Feelings Thermometer rating, the child provides an IR of 2, indicating mild distress and impairment, suggesting that the separation anxiety does not cause them much concern.

To get the most accurate rating possible from the child that signifies the symptom report, when asking for the IR the interviewer should summarize the information gained during the symptom rating section of the diagnostic module as a lead-in to the IR question. For example, *"You've told me that you are very afraid of being in your room alone even in the daytime and of sleeping alone, so you often have your mom sleep with you. You are very afraid of going to a friend's house without your mom, so you don't go on play dates without her. You're also afraid that something bad can happen to you or to your parents if you all aren't together. How much do these problems interfere in your life or mess things up for you?"* This allows the interviewer to summarize for the child what they reported and orient the child to the Feelings Thermometer and allows the child to better consider their response. If the child in the above example still maintains a rating of 2, the clinician records the child's rating and then assigns a Confidence Rating to reflect the discrepancy between the child's endorsement of many symptoms yet their low rating of distress and impairment.

Despite clarifying by summarizing the symptoms endorsed by the child, at times a child will provide an IR that does not reflect their response to the questions within the diagnostic section. For example, a child may have reported significant fear and avoidance of many social situations involving school and peer interactions, but then provides a rating of 3 for overall interference. The interviewer should inquire further and ask the child to give as many examples from their experience as possible to ensure that the child understands the use of the Feelings Thermometer. This is typically sufficient to orient the child to the rating range. If, however, the child continues to stick to what is clearly an invalid rating, the interviewer still reports this as the child's CIR. This is then addressed with a low Confidence Rating, and the interviewer will adjust in the composite (based on combined CIR and PIR) diagnosis and CSR. A note should be made on the ADIS-5 Composite Summary Form (located at the end of the Parent Interview) and on the ADIS-5 Child Interview Summary Form (located at the end of the Child Interview) as to the *confidence* in the diagnosis based upon the child's report (e.g., Confidence Rating would be around 65 in this case, as the minimum number of symptoms is met but the CIR was rated too low). Noting that the child denied interference and distress with a reported rating of 2 should be recorded in the clinical record.

Multiple diagnoses can be present at the same time, and this is not uncommon among the anxiety disorders. If the youth gives the same interference rating for multiple diagnoses, the interviewer should ask at the end of a diagnostic section, "*You had rated your fear of being away from your parents, sleeping alone in your own room, going on overnight sleepovers, and having bad dreams about being away from home as a 6, for how much this messes things up for you. Remember that? Okay, now you've rated fear of water, such as when you're asked to go swimming in a pool for gym class or at the lake during summer, and when you have to be on a ferry, this is also a 6 and messes things up for you with school, friends, and family. Are these two things, being afraid of separating from mom and dad, and being afraid of water, about the same, or is one of these fears worse?*"

Similar to variations in child report, there are times when a parent may rate their child's symptoms and interference as higher or lower than is warranted. For example, a parent may report that their middle school child is hesitant to enter situations with new people, has to be coaxed to call a classmate for missed homework, and expresses some anxiety prior to taking tests. During the interview the parent reports that the child does do all these things, but reluctantly. Assume that the minimum number of symptoms and time frame is met. For the IR, the parent responds with a 7 as the degree of distress and impairment caused by this symptom cluster. Again, the interviewer can review the range of the 0-to-8 scale to ensure the parent understands that higher ratings reflect more severe and impairing disability and distress. An appropriate Confidence Rating and a note should be made on the ADIS Composite Summary Form in relation to the parent's final rating.

## Confidence Ratings

Assign Confidence Ratings (on a scale of 0 = no confidence at all to 100 = completely confident in the diagnosis and CSR) for each identified diagnosis. The Confidence Rating indicates the interviewer's "trust" that the diagnosis and CSR accurately reflect the child's true psychiatric state. Confidence Ratings are lowered by any number of factors, including discrepancies in report, failure to respond to questions, vague or confusing answers, questions about the reporter's (child or parent) cognitive functioning or ability to accurately report information, limited access to certain information (e.g., a parent's inability to know a child's feeling state), inappropriate expectations on the part of the reporter ("I should never feel anxious before a test" or "My 7-year-old child should be comfortable telling the teacher she doesn't make sense to him"), self-presentation biases ("faking bad" or "faking good"), and the nature of certain psychiatric conditions (e.g., fear of negative evaluation associated with social anxiety, inattention, fatigue or withdrawal associated with depression or anxiety, or failure to speak as in selective mutism).

## THE COMPOSITE DIAGNOSIS AND CSR

For the Composite Diagnosis and CSR, combine the information gained during the Child Interview and the Parent Interview with good clinical judgment and knowledge of psychopathology and development. The Composite Diagnosis and CSR are often used as the entry criteria for a clinical trial. Children and parents can differ on their views of symptom presence and severity, along with interference. In the Composite Diagnosis, combine the data following the decision rules outlined below.

**The Composite Diagnosis: Diagnostic Decision Rules**

If only one interview yields a diagnosis, and the CIR and PIR are between 0 and 3, then the CSR for the composite diagnosis is between 0 and 3 (subclinical) and the child does not receive the diagnosis per DSM criteria.*

If one or both interviews yield a diagnosis with an IR $\geq$ 4, the child is assigned the diagnosis at the higher severity rating.

If both interviews yield a diagnosis with a IRs $\geq$4, the child gets the diagnosis at the higher severity rating.

As indicated, the interviewer should use clinical judgment to adjust the CSR for under- or over-reporting by parent or child.

*Note: Clinicians may wish to record a CSR of 0 to 3 to track the course of subclinical symptoms over time.

The ADIS taxonomy for assigned diagnoses is as follows:

1. The *Principal Diagnosis* is the diagnosis with the highest CSR on the Composite Summary Form. There can be co-principal diagnoses, where two or more diagnoses share the same highest level of severity.

2. *Additional Diagnoses* are all other diagnoses for which full criteria are met. These diagnoses would carry CSRs of 4 or greater but would be lesser in severity than the principal one.

3. The ADIS Principal Diagnosis is compared with the term *Primary Diagnosis*, which refers to the diagnosis of earliest onset.

## Operational Definitions (Anchors) for CSR Levels (0–8)

The ADIS CSR is an index of symptom severity and disability. This is not an index of improvement. Thus, at intake, post-treatment evaluations, and any follow-up assessments, the CSR represents the level of severity and disability at the time of the current assessment. It is a snapshot of how the child is functioning at the present time. CSR levels are rendered in comparison to normative levels and levels of severity expressed at the time of evaluation.

Each successive CSR subsumes the behavioral descriptors of the previous level. For example, a child with a diagnosis with a CSR of 6 will likely evidence most or all of the symptoms and disability associated with a CSR of 4, but at a greater intensity, frequency, and/or degree of disability.

1. A CSR of 0 represents that the child is expressing developmentally appropriate and normative, expected levels of anxiety given certain situations (e.g., a little anxiety at the start of school, first oral report, or illness of a family member). This level of anxiety is minimal and transient and dissipates on its own. Again, this is normative anxiety that is experienced by the average child or adolescent.

2. A CSR of 2 represents mild anxiety that is also within the normative and expected range. That is, any child may experience this type of anxiety from time to time. It does not lead to excessive avoidance in any concerning degree and may be associated with minimal or minor distress.

3. A CSR of 3 is approaching clinical significance. At a level of 3, the child is experiencing many symptoms in an anxiety category, but perhaps not all of the symptoms, *or* they are not experiencing significant impairment due to the symptoms, *or* they do not meet the time course required for the diagnosis. This anxiety is "hanging on" longer than the previous levels (0–2) and can still remit on its own, but it may, with time, become worse. Some children may not develop a disorder, even though a level of 3 may be reported during times of stress (e.g., exam periods, parental divorce, illness, peer problems) or developmental change (e.g., transition to a new grade or school, initiation of dating). A level of 3 is usually considered "prodromal" (if the child never had the diagnosis) or "in partial remission" (if there was evidence of the disorder in the recent past, and some symptoms remain). A level of 3 may also indicate a more temperamentally anxious child but not at the level of warranting a diagnosis or clinical intervention. Also, if the ADIS is conducted post-treatment, and the child or adolescent is no longer meeting criteria for a diagnosis, a level of

3 is warranted if the time course to full remission (as defined in DSM-5) is not yet met.

4. A level of 4 represents that the child meets all diagnostic criteria for the disorder and that the anxiety is beyond the range of what is expected and accepted as normal. The child meets all required symptoms, including time course and impairment. This level of anxiety usually involves avoidance and definitely interferes with the child's functioning, as it crosses the threshold to a clinical disorder and is viewed as "just outside the norm." This child is in need of treatment because efforts by the parents or child to resolve the anxiety at home have not worked and the child's anxiety persists.

5. A level of 6 represents that the child meets all diagnostic criteria for the disorder and that the anxiety is well beyond the range of what is expected for the child's age. It is neither appropriate nor normative, and is associated with increasing avoidance and distress. This level indicates significant impairment in functioning. This child should be in treatment and may have failed to respond to prior treatment attempts.

6. A level of 8 represents that "this is the worst level of anxiety (or other disorder, such as depression) for anyone" as the child meets *all* diagnostic criteria for the disorder, the anxiety is extreme for any age, and there is significant impairment and distress. This child is in need of intensive intervention. A CSR of 8 is not given frivolously; these youth evidence extreme impairment in functioning due to the diagnosis in question.

Table 1.1 contains examples of symptoms across these CSRs for the triad of child anxiety disorders: Separation Anxiety Disorder, Social Anxiety Disorder, and GAD.

## OVERVIEW OF DIFFERENTIAL DIAGNOSTIC ISSUES

This section reviews essential differences between certain diagnostic categories but is not a substitute for having a thorough working knowledge of child and adolescent development, psychopathology, and the DSM criteria for mental disorders.

### Differentiating Social Phobia from Panic Disorder

Panic attacks can occur in the context of situations that provoke social anxiety, and the individual with social phobia may experience full- or limited-symptom panic attacks upon the demand for social interaction, performance, or evaluation. However, the fear in social phobia is of the social situation, and the panic attack itself is secondary to (a result of) this fear. In contrast, in Panic Disorder, the fear is of the symptoms of the panic attack itself. The individual will fear these symptoms in any context (e.g., home, school, alone) and not just in social situations.

**TABLE 1.1  Clinician Severity Ratings (CSR)***

CSR = 0: Absence of symptoms/No disturbance in functioning/No disability
Child may express (verbally or noted via observation by others) developmentally appropriate levels of anxiety, fear, or worry at times in response to specific novel or challenging situations. For the most part, the anxiety dissipates spontaneously during the situation. The youth does not avoid the situation or stimulus and is able to function in all spheres (social, academic, family, and self-care) with no disruption or disability.

*Examples:*

| Separation Anxiety Disorder | Social Anxiety Disorder (Social Phobia) | Generalized Anxiety Disorder |
|---|---|---|
| Initial hesitancy to enter a new situation where separation from parents is involved, such as the first days of school, camp, or a first sleepover; parents traveling away for work or vacation without child; staying with a new babysitter; or going away without parents. The child may ask questions about whether the parents will be home in case they are needed and whether they will pick up the child at the end of the event. Initial and expected anxiety associated with such novel separation situations may be expressed in verbal or overt behavior, but habituates quickly and with repeated experience with the task. The child is able to accept a reasonable degree of reassurance and be redirected to the positive aspects of a situation. | Initial hesitancy to enter a new social situation such as the first days of school, camp, or attendance at a party that may be expressed through a "What if" question such as "What if I don't make friends?" or "What if the teacher is mean?" The child is able to accept a reasonable degree of reassurance and be redirected to the positive aspects of a situation. The child "warms up" to the people present, and settles into the situation. | Youth may express (verbally or noted via observation by others) developmentally appropriate levels of concern or worry that are circumscribed to specific events and are brief in duration. Children tend to ask questions that indicate curiosity and worry as they encounter new concepts and situations during development such as "Are you (or grandma, e.g.) going to die?" "Why do you and mom/dad fight? Are you getting a divorce?" The youth is able to be reassured with little to no difficulty, is able to focus on tasks and enjoy themselves, and can completely stop thinking about the concern. There is no distress or avoidance and the child is able to function in all spheres (social, academic, family, and self-care) with no disruption or disability. |

*(continued)*

**TABLE 1.1 Continued**

| Separation Anxiety Disorder | Social Anxiety Disorder (Social Phobia) | Generalized Anxiety Disorder |
|---|---|---|
| A young child is hesitant to stay with a new babysitter or relatively unfamiliar person (even a relative), but after an initial introduction to the person, the child settles and does not remain upset or concerned when the parent exits the situation. | Overt anxious behavior such as standing away from others or hesitancy to initiate conversations or to join an already-formed group may be evident upon entering novel social situations. However, the child becomes engaged upon the invitation of others (adults or peers) or makes their way into the situation with little or no prompting. | Child may express initial concern about new situations or events in the form of a "What if" question, but is able to accept the parents' answer and move on to a new topic. Examples: "What if our first baseball game is rained out?" "What if we can't find a hotel on vacation?" "What if I don't like my teacher this year?" "What if we go to war with another country?" In other words, the child expresses a normal and appropriate level of curiosity about various situations, including academics, world events, safety, and health matters. |
| Child hesitates to sleep alone in a new or unfamiliar situation (e.g., move to "big bed," a new house, at a relative's home, after the arrival of a new sibling); however, with some brief reassurance, the child does sleep alone and through the night. Child may sleep with a nightlight but does not require the parents to stay with them. | This initial hesitancy does not last beyond the first week of encounters of any novel situation (school, camp, move to new neighborhood), given adequate opportunities to socialize or be the focus of attention. | Child or adolescent may be focused on an upcoming event or life situation (e.g., start of school in the fall, upcoming tests, family events) but there is evidence of enthusiasm, coping, or problem solving in relation to the event. For example, the child may answer their own "What if" question and does not appear overly concerned about the event. Instead, there is curiosity or positive/optimistic expectancies associated with the event. |

**TABLE 1.1 Continued**

| Separation Anxiety Disorder | Social Anxiety Disorder (Social Phobia) | Generalized Anxiety Disorder |
|---|---|---|
| Child is hesitant about attending sleepaway camp. They may become upset when being dropped off at camp and may feel homesick for a few days. Child may tell parents that they want to go home. However, once the child becomes engaged in camp activities, they are able to enjoy it and no longer become upset about being away from home. | Child participates in age-appropriate activities such as engaging with peers in play or conversation, ordering food in restaurants, answering the telephone, accepting invitations from peers, asking for help from appropriate adults (e.g., teachers, the parents of other children), responding to questions in class, and offering appropriate responses to verbal stimuli (e.g., says "please" or "thank you"). | In response to real stressors (e.g., a sick relative, final exams), the child is able to accept reassurance and/or a problem-solving plan with help from the parent (or teacher, if a school situation) and move on to other activities as appropriate. |
| Child wants the parent to be present for the initial two or three times of going to an event (e.g., birthday party), but not necessarily to stay at the event for its duration (e.g., parent can leave after 20 minutes). | Initial and expected anxiety associated with performance tasks (e.g., giving an oral report, dance recitals, sports activities, tests) may be expressed in verbal or some overt behavior, but habituates quickly and with repeated experience with the task. | |
| Child is initially hesitant, but then engages in age-appropriate activities such as going to other children's houses, sleepovers, day camp, and staying home with a babysitter or to be alone at home for periods of time. | Adolescents may express initial reluctance or anxiety to engage in age-appropriate developmental tasks such as seeking employment, asking for or accepting a date, requesting clarification on academic tasks from teachers/tutors, increased concern about academic achievement or exams, and nervousness associated with interviews (e.g., college, jobs). This anxiety may be evident but not out of proportion to the demands of the situation, it is short in duration, and it does not prevent the adolescent from engaging in the task. | |

(continued)

**TABLE 1.1 Continued**

| Separation Anxiety Disorder | Social Anxiety Disorder (Social Phobia) | Generalized Anxiety Disorder |
|---|---|---|
| Adolescents express initial reluctance or anxiety to engage in age-appropriate developmental tasks such as an extended class trip (e.g., 1 week) or going away to college. This anxiety may be evident, but not out of proportion to the demands of the situation; it is short in duration and does not prevent the adolescent from engaging in the task. | | |

CSR = 2: Mild symptoms/Slight disturbance in functioning/Not really disabled
Child expresses (verbal or via observation by others) developmentally appropriate levels of anxiety, fear, or worry that are circumscribed to specific events/interactions and brief in duration. The anxiety may not dissipate during the course of the first several situations, but the youth **does not avoid** the situation and is able to function in all spheres (social, academic, family, and self-care) with very minor disruption but no disability. In this case, the child may take several days to a week or need several experiences with the situation before the anxiety habituation is evident.

*Examples:*

| Separation Anxiety Disorder | Social Anxiety Disorder (Social Phobia) | Generalized Anxiety Disorder |
|---|---|---|
| Child expresses reservations about novel separation situations such as a first sleepover or sleeping over at a new friend's house, or going away with a friend's family. The child may need to call the parents before going to sleep at the friend's house and/or wants to bring a security object such as a pillow, blanket, or stuffed animal. The child may be unable to sleep over at the friend's house the first time, but will be successful after no more than four attempts (if below age 12; youth 12 and older are expected to do a sleepover without interruption). | Youth may openly express reservations about a novel or challenging social situation, such as the start of school, camp, or an evaluative/performance situation. The youth may need occasional prompting, encouragement, or reassurance to engage in these tasks for a week to a few months until comfort is achieved. | Child may ask the same or similar questions a number of times about a novel or challenging upcoming situation, as indicative of mild levels of anticipatory anxiety, such as inquiries about plans ("Who is picking us up and from what location?"), risk ("What if I don't pass the entrance exam for the school?"), deadlines ("When is that due again?"), and similar issues or contexts. |

**TABLE 1.1 Continued**

| Separation Anxiety Disorder | Social Anxiety Disorder (Social Phobia) | Generalized Anxiety Disorder |
|---|---|---|
| Parents hear from babysitters that the child wanted to call them and asked for them throughout the evening, but nevertheless, the child goes to sleep and does not wait up for the parents. | Youth does not avoid these situations and is able to function adequately in them (e.g., does engage in conversations with others, gives oral reports) although some anxiety may be evident during the task. Such anxiety may take the form of blushing, shaky voice, poor eye contact, low volume of voice, and delaying the start of the task. | Child or adolescent may display anxiety or worry over situations such as forgetting their homework, misplacing an object, arguments with friends, upcoming report cards, or doctor or dental appointments, but after a short time the child is able to stop the worry and proceed with usual activities. |
| Child expresses some reluctance to go places without the parents (e.g., have another child's parent take them somewhere) but their concern does not stop them from doing the activity. | Youth may need some prompting for situations such as calling friends for play dates or missed homework, ordering their food in restaurants, answering the telephone or returning texts or emails, signing up for performance-based activities, and responding to adult/authority figures. | Child or adolescent does not float from one worry to another; that is, the child is "worry free" for most of the time. |
| Child expresses openly reservations about an extended-separation situation, such as the start of school or camp. The child needs occasional prompting, encouragement, or reassurance for the first few weeks (but no longer than 4–6 weeks) until comfort is achieved. | There is initial hesitancy to advocate for oneself with a teacher or adult supervisor (e.g., ask for an extension on homework or for time off from a job or internship) during the first few times a situation presents itself, but the adolescent does this with prompting. | Child's or adolescent's worries, when they occur, are age-appropriate and short-lived, and do not cause disruption in functioning. |

(continued)

**TABLE 1.1 Continued**

| Separation Anxiety Disorder | Social Anxiety Disorder (Social Phobia) | Generalized Anxiety Disorder |
|---|---|---|
| Child requests that the parents call in to say "good night" when out, but there is little or no protest or request for the parents to come home. In other words, the call satisfies the child and they go to sleep without difficulty. | | Child or adolescent does not worry unnecessarily. There is usually a realistic stressor or event that prompts an expected or normal amount of anxiety. |
| Child or young adolescent uses a nightlight and wants an extended "tuck in" that lasts no more than 15 minutes. The parents are able to opt out of the tuck-in routine with little distress expressed by the child, and the child goes to sleep on their own. | | |
| Child may experience an illness such as the flu or may have been hospitalized due to appendicitis, and asks to sleep with the parent during the episode of illness. This is a transient anxiety state that is not unusual and the child should evidence a return to sleeping alone quite quickly | | |

**TABLE 1.1  Continued**

CSR = 4: Moderate symptoms/Definite disturbance in functioning/Disabling
Child meets full criteria for an anxiety disorder (minimum number of required symptoms) plus evident impairment in one or more contexts (with peers, family, or school/work situations). The child may or may not be able to acknowledge the presence of symptoms or disability, but parents note overt behavioral avoidance of, or anxiety related to, age-appropriate activities and tasks. The child's anxiety remains constant for the required time frame outlined in the DSM-5, with no true abatement of symptoms or disability. That is, despite ongoing opportunities to engage in various challenging situations or with stimuli, the child remains anxious (does not habituate or develop tolerance of discomfort) and may engage in active avoidance of these situations. Moreover, there is evidence for disruption in functioning in one or more domains (self-care, school/work, social relationships, and family functioning).

*Examples:*

| Separation Anxiety Disorder | Social Anxiety Disorder (Social Phobia) | Generalized Anxiety Disorder |
|---|---|---|
| Child expresses reservations concerning engaging in situations outside of the home (e.g., school, birthday parties, play dates, sleepovers, day camp) through either statements of anxiety or overt behavioral indicators such as crying, pleading, delaying, or avoiding the situation. This occurs with each repeat situation and does not diminish in the intensity of upset expressed by the child. | Child may not own up to the social anxiety, but parents note overt behavioral avoidance of, or anxiety related to, age-appropriate activities and tasks that may be circumscribed (e.g., solely focused on tests or oral reports, or other performance situations) or more generalized. In many cases, the parents may note the absence of activity or that the child dropped out of activities (e.g., "No, he does not go to school events," or "She never texts/uses social media/uses the telephone," or "He used to play baseball but won't do that anymore"). | Child or adolescent has a difficult time controlling their worry, and always seems to be worrying about something. They cannot be easily reassured or redirected to another task. Child may be considered a "worrywart," "high-strung," or anxious by others (e.g., teacher, other adults). |

(*continued*)

**TABLE 1.1 Continued**

| Separation Anxiety Disorder | Social Anxiety Disorder (Social Phobia) | Generalized Anxiety Disorder |
|---|---|---|
| Child often checks on where the parent is at home; for example, if the child is playing in one room, they go to check on where the parent is located in the house. | Anxiety and avoidance may result in a lack or loss of friendships, concern expressed by school personnel ("If only she would speak up in class!"), and a failure to act independently in social situations (e.g., separate from family to mingle at outings or social events). | Child frequently asks questions, may repeat a question several times, and is often unable to accept an answer, which leads to continued doubt and worry. |
| Child wants the parent(s) to lay down with them at night until child is asleep. Often, the child goes into the parents; room during the night and, despite being taken back to their own bed, this happens repeatedly. | Child may use excuses for their avoidance of social or evaluative situations, such as blaming the teacher ("She is mean, so I don't want to be in that class") or peers ("I don't go to parties because everyone is doing drugs") or complaining of fears of looking foolish in front of others ("Everyone will laugh at me"). | Child may check and recheck homework, and despite evidence to the contrary, doubts their competency on academic or athletic tasks. |
| Child avoids (or escapes from) going to sleepovers, field trips, weekend retreats, sleepaway camp. If the child is made to go on these activities, the adult supervisors report the child was distressed. Child may be sent home due to being unable to settle into a routine. | Adolescents may express more than "average" concern regarding appearance, competencies (in social skills, school, sports, other performance events), and social stature relative to peers. | Child or adolescent worries about events or situations that have a low likelihood of occurrence, and despite knowing this, continues to worry (e.g., worry about natural disasters, failure despite good grades, parental divorce despite a good marriage). |

**TABLE 1.1 Continued**

| Separation Anxiety Disorder | Social Anxiety Disorder (Social Phobia) | Generalized Anxiety Disorder |
|---|---|---|
| Child may have a tantrum or become angry when parents plan to leave to go out and may repeatedly ask that parents "promise" to be home by a certain time. Child contacts parents several times while they are away from home to "check on them." | The youth may develop a reliance on others to engage in a social situation, such as refusal to enter the cafeteria, attend a party or school event, or return to a camp or athletic/social activity without a trusted friend (i.e., "safety person"). The youth will drop out of or avoid these activities and situations without the person who provides (unknowingly or knowing) support and cover for their anxiety. | Child becomes easily upset and may cry or display anger or tantrum behavior when frustrated with a task (e.g., losing a game, solving a homework problem); this type of behavior happens often, as the child has little tolerance for less-than-perfect performance or any perceived failure. |
| Anxiety and avoidance may result in a lack or loss of friendships because the child is missing age-appropriate social events (i.e., sleepovers) and exhibiting poor school performance because the child is distracted by the anxiety while at school. | A repeated habit of missing school or activities at times when there is an expected performance or when the youth will be the focus of attention is evident to others. Such avoidance may entail missing school on exam or oral report days, dropping out of camp/other structured extracurricular activity prior to a performance (e.g., camp play; choral, dance, or musical instrument recital), dropping out of sports teams or chess, math, or robotics clubs prior to tournaments or before the event, and similar situations. | Child may appear clingy or needy, in that they are constantly seeking reassurance and validation from parents ("Is that okay, mom?"), peers ("Are you mad at me? Are we best friends?"), or teachers ("Did I get that right?"). In fact, the child may wind up being rejected by peers due to this type of neediness, and teachers may want to impose an intervention if the child is constantly in need of attention and reassurance. |

*(continued)*

**TABLE 1.1 Continued**

| Separation Anxiety Disorder | Social Anxiety Disorder (Social Phobia) | Generalized Anxiety Disorder |
|---|---|---|
| The child uses excuses such as saying it is "more fun at home" and that it is "boring" to go places outside of the home in an attempt to avoid leaving home and parents. The child may express wishes to have friends come over rather than go to others' houses. | Child or adolescent expresses anxiety and upset in relation to future social or evaluative situations, and cannot be reassured or engage in constructive problem solving or planning. | Child has difficulty with group activities and projects because of an inability to delegate or share responsibility ("No one cares as much as I do" or "The other kids don't do as good a job as I can"). This may cause problems with peers, but more likely, it causes added and undue stress for the youth who cannot fully enjoy a group activity. |
| Adolescent may express a desire to stay with parents that is excessive for their developmental level, and report too much worry when there is an opportunity to be away from home (e.g., attend a sleepover), so they choose to stay around the house. | | Child's or adolescent's worries continue despite natural breaks in routine. That is, the child worries about school during the holidays or summer vacation, or worries about their next developmental hurdle (e.g., Will I get into a good college?) despite the event being in the distant future. |
| Older adolescents may become upset or angry when talk of leaving home for college or travel (e.g., school trips or other travel without parents) occurs, and the youth actively avoids planning for these situations. | | Reassurance or the conclusion of a stressful period does not result in lasting comfort for the child or adolescent. In effect, the child or adolescent does not take time off from their worry. They always appear to be looking for the next problem or struggle. |

**TABLE 1.1 Continued**

CSR = 6: Severe symptoms/Marked disturbance in functioning/Markedly disabling
Child exhibits increasing distress and disability that interferes markedly with functioning in several domains. Child may be exhibiting school refusal behavior; stable patterns of avoidance of anxiety- or fear-provoking situations in several areas; and decreased functioning in usual, non–anxiety-related activities (e.g., activities of daily living, age-appropriate play or leisure activity, interest in events and situations in the child's family and community). Child may exhibit a lack of response to a monotherapy or increasing noncompliance with therapy, such that multimodal therapy is initiated or under consideration. Comorbid mood and behavioral symptoms may be emerging. The child may also be falling behind their same-age peers in typical developmental tasks for their age (e.g., activities of daily living such as self-care or care of personal belongings; ability to manage age-appropriate tasks such as feeding self, preparing snacks or meals, choosing a self-directed activity for enjoyment, or taking on tasks such as completing applications, learning to drive, and similar age-related activity).

*Examples:*

| Separation Anxiety Disorder | Social Anxiety Disorder (Social Phobia) | Generalized Anxiety Disorder |
|---|---|---|
| Child is unable to separate from parents during the evaluation and demands that at least one parent sit with them during the ADIS. If this is not accommodated, child may be upset and ask repeatedly to see the parents. The child or teen engages in active attempts to avoid separation from parents/home via hiding from parents, feigning illness, crying/begging parents, or having tantrums. | Conversations with others (peers or adults) may be difficult and the youth's social behaviors may be misunderstood as poor social skills (e.g., poor eye contact, low voice volume, hanging hair in front the eyes, failure to acknowledge others who address the youth). | Child or adolescent may struggle more often than not with academic tasks, performance activities (e.g., playing games, dance, sports) due to fear of failing at a self-imposed, high standard. The child "stresses" over getting things right or perfect, so much so that performance may actually be impaired. |
| Child's avoidance of activities (e.g., birthday parties, sleepovers) increases to a near-constant or steady frequency and is accompanied by much distress and upset. Child is typically fine with having friends visit at their home, so it is not the activity itself or peers, but it is the separation that is problematic. Consequently, child's social life centers on their home. All play dates and sleepovers take place at the child's house as there is unwillingness to go to other's homes. | Child engages in active attempts to avoid social situations (e.g., school, friendships, evaluative situations, parties) and succeeds in avoidance more times than not. Distress is evident through either statements of anxiety or overt behavioral indicators such as crying, pleading, delaying, leaving, or avoiding the situation. | Child or adolescent has difficulty relaxing and enjoying non-evaluative, leisure activities. Crying, tantrums, or withdrawal may occur in response to being directed to "relax and have fun." These children are unable to soothe or calm themselves. |

*(continued)*

**TABLE 1.1 Continued**

| Separation Anxiety Disorder | Social Anxiety Disorder (Social Phobia) | Generalized Anxiety Disorder |
|---|---|---|
| Child has significant difficulty attending school or day camp. This causes significant family conflict almost every morning prior to school or camp. The child may need to be escorted into school by parent or school counselor. The parent may feel the need to stay at school for some time each day until the child feels comfortable, but this *does not get better* over time. School or camp personnel report the child's separation-related upset causes problems for other participants and the staff. Youth at this level of severity may be missing school more days than not due to the separation anxiety. They receive a lot of attention for this problem. | Some youth may develop certain rationalizations for their isolation, such as "Other kids my age are immature," "My hobbies/ interests are different from others," "I don't enjoy parties and similar social events," "All the kids in my class do drugs and I don't want to be exposed to that." This is a gross overgeneralization to compensate for feelings of loneliness and isolation. | Peers or family members may not like to play with this child because they are "bossy" or too tense. The child is not appropriately assertive in play but is pushy in trying to get playmates to conform to some standard that may be unattainable. |
| Child is constantly demanding to be with the parent(s) and will refuse to play alone in one room of the house while the parent(s) is in another. | Youth at this level may have created a self-contained "world" at home, consisting of a certain hobby or interest that is exclusive of others and replaces social interaction, or participates solely in activity that does not require face-to-face social contact (e.g., online gaming). Often, the youth appears "fine" with this solitary activity (cf., "ego-syntonic") and verbalizes a preference for this over social interaction. | Child has great difficulty with group academic tasks, as other youth are seen as "not as smart or good" and unable to contribute to the project. The youth will then micromanage the activity, adding undue stress and anxiety and potentially alienating peers over time. |

**TABLE 1.1 Continued**

| Separation Anxiety Disorder | Social Anxiety Disorder (Social Phobia) | Generalized Anxiety Disorder |
| --- | --- | --- |
| Parents rarely go out without the child and have severely limited their social interactions with other adults. This is a result of the child disrupting the parents' activities when out (e.g., repeated phone calls begging the parents to come home; extensive crying and tantrums if parents try to leave home). | Youth may complain of loneliness and isolation but not engage in overt attempts to meet others. | Child or adolescent needs constant reassurance and comforting by others. |
| Child asks to carry a mobile phone to contact parents numerous times during the school day or other separations. This is excessive and unnecessary (i.e., parent went out to grocery store for 30 minutes and child called two or three times to check when parent was coming home). | Family conflict occurs, unless the parents themselves are socially anxious, centering on the adolescent's inability or unwillingness to engage in age-appropriate activities. | Disruption in functioning is mounting, as the child appears fixated on various worries and has difficulty talking about anything but these concerns. |
| Child reports rationalizations for wanting to stay at home, such as "Other kids' houses are boring," "I need to stay at home to keep you [parents] from getting lonely," "I am at school all week; I want to stay home on the weekends to spend time with you [parents]," "It would be better for me to do online schooling." | Anxiety and avoidance have resulted in a lack or loss of friendships, concern expressed by school personnel due to not meeting standards in academic activities, and reluctance to engage in social situations even with the family. | Academic and social behaviors are very impaired due to the anxiety. For example, this child spends an inordinate amount of time on academic tasks, or frets needlessly over leisure and play activities, ultimately resulting in performance deficits in these areas. |

*(continued)*

**TABLE 1.1 Continued**

CSR = 8: Very severe symptoms/Very severe disturbance in functioning/Very severely disabling
Child meets full criteria for an anxiety disorder (minimum number of required symptoms) plus extreme impairment in *several or all* areas of functioning. Child is at the level of severity that warrants intensive intervention, especially if comorbid conditions exist, and programs such as day treatment, intensive outpatient, and inpatient or residential programs are appropriate for consideration. Child may continue to deny the presence of symptoms or disability; however, these symptoms are readily apparent to others just by observation. The anxiety is evident, stable, and disabling, and child may have not responded to one or more attempts at treatment with monotherapy or multimodal therapy. Child actively avoids most situations and stimuli that provoke anxiety and is likely refusing to attend school. Disruption in functioning is evident and significant as the child may have no friendships or an inability to initiate and/or maintain friends, and possible academic problems (some stemming from school refusal). There is likely to be family conflict secondary to the anxiety disorder. This child or adolescent may be lagging significantly behind same-age peers in typical development and is falling behind on emerging self-identity and self-awareness, life-management skills, short- and long-term academic and vocational goals, engagement in home and community activities, and progress with developing and deepening relationships with others.

*Examples:*

| Separation Anxiety Disorder | Social Anxiety Disorder (Social Phobia) | Generalized Anxiety Disorder |
|---|---|---|
| Child is unable to separate from parent, except in very circumscribed, familiar situations (i.e., stays with a relative for a brief duration of a few hours). | Youth at this level may display active levels of avoidance during the interview as characterized by a refusal to answer questions or will provide only very brief responses. Youth may request to leave the room. Of note may be non-responsiveness to humor or other attempts by the interviewer to engage the youth. In effect, youth at this level may be very difficult to interview and are noticeably uncomfortable with the situation. | Child or adolescent has great difficulty with independent functioning, and rarely makes decisions on their own. Thinking is characterized by excessive doubting and rumination, as the child is unable to render a simple decision without undue worry and anxiety. |

**TABLE 1.1 Continued**

| Separation Anxiety Disorder | Social Anxiety Disorder (Social Phobia) | Generalized Anxiety Disorder |
|---|---|---|
| Child or teen refuses to attend school on a daily basis; as a result, parents may have given in to home schooling (or online schooling) or child is receiving tutoring at home. | Conversations with others (peers or adults) rarely occur as these are difficult and experienced as painful for the youth. Youth with anxiety at this level of intensity rarely interact with others in situations such as talking on the telephone, using social media, texting, accepting play dates or party invitations, or asking for help. Essentially, youth at this level have "micro" encounters of very brief interaction, which are experienced as distressing. | Parents (and potentially the teacher) are providing constant reassurance and supervision of the child or adolescent in most areas of functioning. |
| Child or adolescent attempts to sleep with parent(s) or a sibling almost every night to feel safe. There is excessive disruption and distress around the sleeping situation. | Adolescents are clearly overly concerned about appearance, competencies (in social skills, school, sports, other performance events), and social stature relative to what is typical for same-aged peers. However, the adolescent may not be able to report these concerns to either a family member or professional. Some adolescents will report feeling less competent or attractive than peers, and talk about themselves consistently in self-deprecating ways. | Child may be unable to attend school due to constant worry, rumination, inability to focus attention and complete tasks, and overall fear. |

*(continued)*

**TABLE 1.1 Continued**

| Separation Anxiety Disorder | Social Anxiety Disorder (Social Phobia) | Generalized Anxiety Disorder |
|---|---|---|
| Child or adolescent rarely leaves the parent(s), even in their own home, and only for brief durations (e.g., to take a bath). | Parents will describe the youth as "always like this" but perhaps "getting even worse." Youth at this level have typically suffered with a lifelong and stable inhibition that has increased in intensity over time to social anxiety disorder. These children are often described as "painfully shy," "loners," or "isolates." | Due to the extreme nature of the worry, the differential diagnosis of GAD from OCD (worry rumination versus obsessions) or from ADHD (the concentration impairment or physiological reactivity due to worry or the externalizing condition) may be difficult. A careful review of the DSM criteria is necessary as are understandings of the developmental trajectories of each disorder. |
| Child complains of safety fears (will be kidnapped or someone will break in to the house; parents may be killed) even in extremely unlikely situations (e.g., family lives on 25th floor of a building with 24-hour security guards). | Child may complain of loneliness and isolation. However, some youth at this level of distress may appear avoidant and express (upon questioning) a desire to be alone. | |
| Child avoids all situations requiring separation from parents. Any situations that the child does attend, such as school or allowing a parent to leave home for errands, likely occur because child is "dragged" to the situation or coerced/bribed by parents. | Adolescents with this level of intensity of social anxiety find it difficult to think or talk about future plans, such as college, career, and relationships, due to the fear of interacting with others. | |
| Child remains distressed during any separation situation and may become physically aggressive when forced to separate. | | |
| Adolescents fail to separate for age-appropriate tasks such as school trips, vacations with friends, college visits, and similar separation activities. | | |

*Note: Each successive level of severity subsumes all of the criteria from the previous level.

*Social Phobia*

1. Panic attacks are cued by social situations.
2. Avoided situations always involve other people.
3. Main fear is of negative evaluation, embarrassment, rejection, humiliation.

*Panic Disorder*

1. Panic attacks occur spontaneously.
2. Situations are avoided whether or not others are involved.
3. Main fear is of the symptoms of panic: Something is physically wrong with me!

## Differentiating Social Phobia from GAD

The differential diagnosis of Social Phobia from GAD can be troublesome due to shared symptoms and contexts. Youth with Social Phobia worry about their performance, friendships, school, and other matters, and this often results in the quandary of "which diagnosis fits the child or teenager best?" We offer some general guidelines for this diagnostic distinction. If the worry occurs solely in the presence or anticipated presence of others, due to fear of negative evaluation, then Social Phobia is warranted. For example, if a child reports worry about homework, but the worry is solely focused on impressing the teacher, then Social Phobia is warranted. If, however, the focus is on the homework being counted toward the overall grade, and the child fears that they will fail the class, then GAD is more likely warranted. Social Phobia is associated with fear of not meeting the standards set by others (not being good enough, not being liked well enough, not pleasing certain adults), whereas GAD is often associated with self-imposed standards (failing to beat a personal best or having high standards for oneself).

*Social Phobia*

1. Worry is focused on performance and social/evaluative situations.
2. The anxiety dissipates upon avoidance or escape of the situation.
3. The anxiety and avoidance may interfere with the child's ability to make or keep friendships. Focus is on what other people think.

*GAD*

1. Worry is on areas other than just performance or interpersonal.
2. The worry does not stop, even with active avoidance or escape.
3. Friendships are not typically avoided.
4. Focus is usually on a self-imposed, unrealistic standard.

### Differentiating Panic Disorder from GAD

Similar to the distinction for Panic Disorder and Social Phobia, youth with GAD may experience panic attacks when excessively worried. However, the physiological responses characteristic of GAD include a state of tension and anxious apprehension, as opposed to the classic fight-or-flight response found in panic attacks and Panic Disorder.

*Panic Disorder*

1. The fight-or-flight response predominates, with increased heart rate, dizziness, shortness of breath, and/or other panic attack symptoms being the focus of concern.
2. The symptoms themselves cause fear and/or avoidance.
3. The panic dissipates upon avoidance or escape from the situation.

*GAD*

1. The child may experience physical tension, apprehension, irritability, fatigue, or other symptoms of stress.
2. The anxiety and worry continue despite avoidance or escape of situations.

### Differentiating Panic Disorder from Separation Anxiety Disorder

Much has been written about whether there exists a developmental progression of Separation Anxiety Disorder into Panic Disorder. This question remains without a definitive answer, but it is well known that these disorders share certain features. For one, in both disorders there is a fear of being alone and left without a trusted person to offer help in the event of an untoward event. Excessive anxiety is present, and often the individual with SAD or panic will shrink away from activities outside of the home. There are, however, essential differences to these disorders that are summarized below.

*Panic Disorder*

1. Symptoms of the fight-or-flight response result in panic attacks that seem to come from "out of the blue" and are not prompted by any situation or thought.
2. The symptoms themselves cause fear and/or avoidance.
3. The panic may dissipate upon avoidance or escape from the situation.
4. A "safety person" is there to stop panic or assist when panic occurs.

*Separation Anxiety Disorder*

1. Main somatic complaints are headaches or stomachaches, not the physical sensations of panic.

2. Focus of fear is separation, not physical symptoms.

3. Fear is of loss of or separation from loved ones, not for the sake of safety from physical symptoms.

## Additional Questions and Suggested Probes

The following section provides additional ways to question children, adolescents, and parents during the course of the ADIS interview. These questions are intended as a guide for the interviewer and should be used to probe further into understanding the intensity, frequency, and duration of the child's anxiety, in addition to gathering information to assess the developmental appropriateness, impact, and context within which the anxiety occurs.

### Interviewing the Youth

Additional probes for children and adolescents:

1. *What would make this situation easier for you?*

2. *Is there anything you do, or anyone you need to have with you, to help you feel less scared? What/Who?*

3. *Are there times when you can (stay home alone, stand up and give a talk, not worry so much)? Tell me about those times.*

4. *What makes that (situation, person, place, thing) scary for you?*

5. *What do you think will happen if you stay (in the situation/with the person)?*

6. *How would your life be different if you weren't worried/scared/anxious?*

7. *If grades didn't matter, would you still worry about school? What would you worry about?*

### Interviewing the Parents

It is preferable to interview both parents at the same time; *however, the primary caregiver should always be interviewed.* If there is a discrepancy between parent responses, note the differing views as it may indicate differential responses from the child in relation to family dynamics. We have also found that using the Feelings Thermometer with parents is helpful for anchoring their responses and ratings.

*Additional Questions for Parents: Social Phobia*

1. *Who orders for your child/teen in restaurants?*

2. *Does your child/teen call/text/email classmates for missed homework?*

3. *Does your child/teen socialize with relatives?*

4. *Is your teen able to make purchases or exchange/return goods on their own?*

5. *What are your child/teen's telephone, text, and social media habits?*

6. *How often does your child/teen do things with peers outside of school and face to face with others (not online)?*

7. *Does your child/teen eat in front of others?*

8. *Does your child/teen participate in any sports or clubs? If not, or if they have stopped these activities, why?*

9. *Do you think you and your teen have the same struggles as other families with an adolescent? What is different than others?*

10. *If (certain situation) did not involve other people, would your child/teen be more comfortable?*

*Additional Questions for Parents: Separation Anxiety Disorder*

1. *Are there times when your child is able to (be alone, stay with a sitter)? When? What is happening then? How often?*

2. *How has this problem interfered with your life? What do you or your spouse/family do differently because of this anxiety?*

3. *What makes things better for your child?*

4. *When your child is upset over (a separation anxiety disorder situation), what are you thinking and feeling?*

*Additional Questions for Parents: GAD*

1. *What have you found that works to help your child calm down or stop worrying?*

2. *How much help do you give your child (with homework, etc.)? Do you think this is too little, enough, or too much?*

3. *How much time does it take your child to do (homework, chores, self-care)?*

4. *What keeps your child from doing things efficiently?*

*Additional Questions for Parents: Anxiety Disorders*

1. *How do/would other people describe your child (teachers, relatives, other adults)?*

2. *In what way would you like to see your child be more independent/self-reliant?*

3. *What does your child do to soothe or calm themselves?*

4. *How long can your child go without being anxious/worried?*

# SUPPLEMENTAL SERVICES ADIS MODULE

This optional section is provided to gather information pertaining to any clinical evaluations or services delivered outside of your practice setting.

Patient ID:_____          Evaluator:_____

Location:_____

Date:_____

Person(s) supplying information (check all that apply):

___Mother     ___Father     ___Child/Teen

___Other (e.g., legal guardian; specify:_____)

Evaluation at:

_____Intake_____ Week 12_____ Week 24_____ Week 36

_____ Other (specify:_____)

For first-time interviews: **Has your child received any of the following services?**

For follow-up assessments: **Since your last interview** (or, concurrent with services from this clinic), **has your child received any of the following services:**

I. <u>Evaluation or diagnostic consultation</u> for anxiety, depression, or other emotional or behavioral **difficulties** (be sure to inquire for family problems, somatic complaints, divorce-custody issues, school adjustment problems):

        Yes_____          No_____

If "yes" obtain the following information:

| Type of evaluation (e.g., educational evaluation, medication consult) | Evaluator's name | Reason for evaluation | Date | Recommendations |
|---|---|---|---|---|
|  |  |  |  |  |
|  |  |  |  |  |

| | | | | |
|---|---|---|---|---|
| | | | | |
| | | | | |
| | | | | |
| | | | | |

**II.** <u>Medications</u> for anxiety, depression, ADHD, somatic complaints, or other emotional or behavioral difficulties:

Yes_____          No_____

If "yes" obtain the following information:

| Medication name | Prescribing clinician | Reason for Rx | Start date/End date | Highest dose | Response: Note any adverse side effects |
|---|---|---|---|---|---|
| | | | | | |
| | | | | | |
| | | | | | |
| | | | | | |
| | | | | | |

**III. <u>Psychotherapy or counseling</u> for anxiety, depression, or other emotional or behavioral difficulties** (be sure to inquire for family problems, divorce-custody issues, school adjustment problems; inquire about school counselor visits):

Yes_____          No_____

If "yes" obtain the following information:

| Type of therapy (e.g., family therapy, play therapy, CBT, day treatment, intensive outpatient program, telehealth, electronic or web-based therapy) | Therapist's name (or program name if electronic) | Reason for therapy | Start date/End date | Frequency (e.g., 1x wk; daily) | Response |
|---|---|---|---|---|---|
|  |  |  |  |  |  |
|  |  |  |  |  |  |
|  |  |  |  |  |  |
|  |  |  |  |  |  |
|  |  |  |  |  |  |
|  |  |  |  |  |  |
|  |  |  |  |  |  |

If child or family received telehealth or electronic/internet/web-based treatment, inquire for the frequency of any face-to-face or telehealth sessions with a live therapist that may have been all or part of the program. Note the reason for the telehealth treatment (e.g., due to public health concerns such as the COVID virus outbreak, refusal of the child to attend live sessions, transportation issues or related logistics such as distance).

**IV.** <u>**Hospitalization or residential placement**</u> **for anxiety, depression, or other emotional or behavioral difficulties** (e.g., school refusal, eating disorders, suicidality, child abuse, emergency placements):

       **Yes_____**          **No_____**

If "yes" obtain the following information:

| Type of placement (hospital, residential center, group home) | Facility name | Reason for placement | Start date/End date | Treatment modality | Response |
|---|---|---|---|---|---|
|  |  |  |  |  |  |
|  |  |  |  |  |  |
|  |  |  |  |  |  |
|  |  |  |  |  |  |
|  |  |  |  |  |  |

**V. <u>Support groups</u> for anxiety, depression, or other emotional or behavioral difficulties** (be sure to inquire for grief/loss, divorce support groups, school adjustment problems, social skills, peer problems):

**Yes**_____ **No**_____

If "yes" obtain the following information:

| Type of group (e.g., grief, divorce, social skills) | Leader's degree/sponsor (e.g., CHADD, hospice, school) | Reason for group | Start date/End date | Frequency (e.g., 1x wk) | Response |
|---|---|---|---|---|---|
|  |  |  |  |  |  |
|  |  |  |  |  |  |
|  |  |  |  |  |  |
|  |  |  |  |  |  |
|  |  |  |  |  |  |

**Besides these questions that I just asked, has your child seen a counselor, doctor, or any other person for help with feeling anxious, sad, or other kinds of feelings?**

If "yes," **When was that? Who did you** (your child) **see?**

Include additional clarification or comments from inquiries in space below.

_____

_____

_____

_____

## ADIS CHILD DEVELOPMENTAL AND CLINICAL TIMELINE: PARENT VERSION

To guide the clinical case conceptualization and for treatment planning, the Developmental and Clinical Timeline (Figure 1.1) provides a summary form to capture dates of symptom and disorder onset, setting and environmental events, interventions, and overall course of development.

The following material is provided to guide the clinician's completion of the Developmental and Clinical Timeline based on child and parent report, and completion of the ADIS Supplemental Services Module. A sample of a completed timeline is included in Figure 1.2.

### Developmental and Educational Milestones

Chart the completion of major developmental steps from infancy through late adolescence, and mark off educational milestones and any implementation of accommodations or notes concerning changes in educational or developmental functioning. Table 1.2 lists several milestones. Clinicians should inquire for the range of milestones noted across development.

Life Events
and
Medical
Conditions

Interventions:
Psychotherapy
Medical
Educational

Onset of
Symptoms
and
Disorders

Developmental
and
Educational
Milestones

Along this line, mark 0 to 36 months (0, 6, 12, 18, 24, 30, 36), then after, continue
w/ages 4 through 18

**FIGURE 1.1.** Developmental and Clinical Timeline.

# Developmental and Clinical Timeline

**Life Events and Medical Conditions**

2 yo pneumonia · 3½ high fevers · 3 = Brother born · 4 yo - Hay fever · +virus · +Headaches · 5 = sister born · 6 yo strep · F = dx Cancer · tx c̄ chemo to remission · PGM dies · 7 move to new house

**Interventions: Psychotherapy / Medical / Educational**

5 yo Play tx 1x/wk · 6 yo Play tx 2x/wk · Rx [ Zoloft - AEs · 8 yo - FLX 20mgs · 8 yo EX/RP "too much" Back to play tx · 9:yo EX/RP c̄ CBT therapist good result - STOPPED @ 10 · 11 40 - relapse

**Onset of Symptoms and Disorders**

6 mos: some mel+downs if frustrated · 2 yrs: cried alot on separation · 3-4: irritability just right! · 1: repeating · 3 - tantrums ✗✗ · 4 = "Let me do it alone" · Controls play · 4 = everything in rows · 6 = no regard for authority - Defiant · No friends by 1st grade · 6 = tics · 3rd - bullied · 8 rituals · ↑ meltdowns · Lots of checking · School refusal · 10 yo - made friends @ new school then lost 2° · OC sxs by 11

**Developmental and Educational Milestones**

(40 wk gestation, no problems pre) · 8 lbs · easy baby · milestones on target · age 2: full sentence · [ Pre + K in same school ] · [ School #1 ] · 1st - 5th grade ][ School #2 ]

BIRTH  1  2  3  4  5  — AGE —  6  7  8  9  10  11  ↑ Present

Along this line, mark 0 to 36 months (0, 6, 12, 18, 24, 30, 36), then after, continue w/ages 4 through 18

**FIGURE 1.2.** Sample of a completed Developmental and Clinical Timeline.

**TABLE 1.2  Key Milestones to Record**

| Infancy and Early Childhood (through age 6) | Middle Childhood (through age 13 or end of middle school) | Adolescence/Emerging Adult (through age 18 and end of high school) |
| --- | --- | --- |
| Held head up | Soothes self in the moment when upset | Advocates for self (e.g., with peers, teachers, supervisors) |
| Sat up and stood unassisted | Asks for help when needed | Works independently on academic tasks |
| Walked unassisted | Seeks and initiates activities with others | Seeks advice on own (e.g., college counselor, career advisor) |
| Put several words together | Entertains self when alone or others are not available | Maintains friendships |
| Named objects | Initiates friendships | Seeks volunteer positions/ engages in community service |
| Spoke in sentences | Seeks social activity | Pursues hobby/interests on own |
| Weaned | Increasingly independent in self-care (bathing, dressing on own) | Seeks grooming appointments (barber/hairdresser) on own |
| Slept through the night | Completes chores without much prompting | Shops for own clothing and supplies (e.g., grooming needs, school supplies) |
| Soothed self upon awakening | Able to make or access basic snacks and meal items on own (e.g., gets own drink when thirsty; prepares a basic sandwich for lunch; finds own snacks as appropriate) | Prepares meals for self, including basic cooking |
| Used age-appropriate utensils to feed self | Does sleepovers at friends' homes | Can place orders for food or supplies over the phone or online |
| Reported preferences for clothing | Attends day camp or regular activity during summer outside of the home | Seeks employment (part or full time as appropriate) |
| Separated appropriately for sitters or day care | Entered elementary school; began middle school (grade 5 or 6) | Attends regular medical and dental appointments on own |
| Became fully toilet trained (day and night) | Able to go away to camp or other school or organized sleepaway activity | Manages own medication (taking as prescribed, on time, requests refills) |

(continued)

**TABLE 1.2 Continued**

| Infancy and Early Childhood (through age 6) | Middle Childhood (through age 13 or end of middle school) | Adolescence/Emerging Adult (through age 18 and end of high school) |
|---|---|---|
| Showed interest in others (children, adults) | Able to seek help when feeling ill | Uses debit or credit card appropriately |
| Engaged in reciprocal play (with children, adults) | Completes homework without prompting | Seeks information on next steps (e.g., college search, job/internship openings) and uses advisors appropriately |
| Entered day care, preschool, kindergarten | Seeks intellectual stimulation (e.g., reading, science projects, inquires about current events, asks questions to increase knowledge) | Completes applications on time (e.g., college, job, internship, financial aid) |
| Resolved early childhood, age-appropriate fears (strangers, dark, noise, small animals, separation) | Engages in a hobby or sport activity outside of school | Uses transportation services on own (e.g., public transportation, taxi, or car service) |
| Knows difference between real and imaginary situations/figures | Engages with teachers without parental involvement (e.g., asks for help or clarification; seeks mentoring on extracurricular or academic activities) | Able to travel unaccompanied to distant location |
| Understands the difference between right and wrong; truth versus lie | Involved in school clubs or other school-based, non-academic activity (e.g., sports team, yearbook, choir, student council) | Makes own travel arrangements (including sleeping as well as travel) |
| | Knows and begins to manage own medication schedule and dosing with little prompting | Soothes self when upset; seeks appropriate guidance when needed |
| | Interested in romantic relationships | Obtains a driver's license |
| | Able to shop for own clothing and personal needs | Engages in romantic interests |
| | Uses money responsibly | |
| | Awakes and gets ready for day alone (e.g., using alarm clock) | |

## Onset of Symptoms and Disorders

Note the first onset of symptoms of mental health and behavioral conditions, and age at which DSM criteria were first met. This section also allows the clinician to chart periods of recovery and relapse, and the onset of secondary and comorbid conditions.

The following are suggested abbreviations for charting clinical conditions. Some of these are shown in Figure 1.2:

| SAD | Separation Anxiety Disorder | OCD | Obsessive-Compulsive Disorder |
|---|---|---|---|
| SoP | Social Anxiety | PTSD | Posttraumatic Stress Disorder |
| GAD | Worry, Generalized Anxiety Disorder | ADHD | Attention-Deficit/Hyperactivity Disorder |
| SP | Specific Phobia | DEP | Depression |
| SM | Selective Mutism | Elim | Enuresis/Encopresis |
| AG | Agoraphobia | DIS | Disruptive behavior, defiance |
| PA | Panic attack | SUB | Substance use/abuse |
| PD | Panic Disorder | ODD | Oppositional Defiant Disorder |
| ED | Eating Disorder | CD | Conduct Disorder |
| WK(s) | Week(s) | TX/Rx | Treatment/Prescription |
| MO(s) | Month(s) | 2° | Secondary to |
| YR(s) | Year(s) | DX | Diagnosis |
| SRT | Sertraline | FLX | Fluoxetine (Prozac) |
| BZ | Benzodiazepine | AEs | Adverse events |
| EX/RP | Exposure plus response prevention | DBT | Dialectical behavioral therapy |
| EX | Exposure therapy | CBT | Cognitive behavioral therapy |
| OT | Occupational therapy | PT | Physical therapy |
| SpTX | Speech therapy | FamTx | Family therapy |
| F | Father | M | Mother |
| PGF | Paternal grandfather | MGF | Maternal grandfather |
| PGM | Paternal grandmother | MGF | Paternal grandfather |
| Br | Brother | Sis | Sister |

## Interventions

In this section, note the engagement in and response to psychotherapy and medication for mental health and behavioral conditions. Also, note the use of therapeutics, including occupational therapy, physical therapy, tutoring, alternative schooling, day treatment, residential, and other modalities addressing mental health, developmental, and educational issues. On the Developmental and Clinical Timeline, record response to interventions, including titration of or change in medication. This information may be obtained via the Supplemental Services Module either by having the parent complete the form on their own or via questioning.

## Life Events and Medical Conditions

Inquire about and record key events in the life of the child, including moves of schools and home; change in family structure due to births, divorce, and deaths; the child's awards and achievements; medical illnesses in the child or primary family members; and related life events that occur in the community that may have impacted the child.

# CHAPTER 2

## ANXIETY AND RELATED DISORDERS INTERVIEW SCHEDULE FOR DSM-5, CHILD AND PARENT VERSION: AUTISM SPECTRUM ADDENDUM (ADIS/ASA)

*Connor M. Kerns, Wendy K. Silverman, and Anne Marie Albano*

## OVERVIEW

The ADIS/ASA is a version of the ADIS Parent Interview designed to facilitate differential diagnosis and assessment of anxiety and obsessive-compulsive disorders (OCD) in children on the autism spectrum. The ADIS/ASA assesses for OCD as well as Separation Anxiety Disorder, Social Anxiety Disorder (Social Phobia), Generalized Anxiety Disorder (GAD), and Specific Phobia. In addition, the ADIS/ASA queries for distinct expressions of anxiety that also commonly arise in children on the autism spectrum, such as anxiety associated with sensory sensitivities, executive functioning differences (e.g., difficulties shifting attention), repetitive and restricted behaviors, emotion recognition deficits, social immaturity, and theory-of-mind deficits.

## INTERVIEW STRUCTURE

- The ADIS/ASA follows the basic structure of the ADIS-5-C/P and should be administered according to manual specifications.

- For each module in which sufficient symptoms are endorsed, parents provide a Parent Interference Rating (PIR) to describe the level of interference associated with the reported anxiety symptoms (see pp. 7–10 on Interference Ratings in Chapter 1).

- As in the standard ADIS protocol, PIR, symptom ratings, differential diagnosis guidelines, and items are then used by clinicians to assign a Clinician Severity Rating (CSR), ranging from 0 (No Impairment) to 8 (Severe Impairment), with 4 representing the minimum interference required to support a diagnosis or the presence of clinically significant anxiety problems. (See pp. 10–12 on CSR in Chapter 1.)

- In the ADIS/ASA, PIR and CSR are collected for both DSM-5 anxiety disorder modules and the other variants of anxiety that arise in Autism Spectrum Disorder (ASD).

- The first half of the ADIS/ASA interview gathers basic information about the child's developmental and intervention history (Sections 1–3) as well as details about their autism, cognitive functioning, and social functioning that will inform your subsequent assessment of their anxiety (Section 4). Specifically, this section includes items related to the child's:
  - Social interest, social opportunity, history of social rejection, and social awareness to inform assessment of Social Anxiety Disorder (see pp. 50–52 in this manual)

- Perseverative thinking to aid in the assessment of cognitive inflexibility versus GAD (see pp. 50–52 in this manual)

- Sensory sensitivity to aid in the differential diagnosis of Specific Phobia and sensory aversions (see pp. 50–52 in this manual)

- The second half of the interview (Sections 5–12) assesses DSM-5 anxiety disorders and distinct expressions of anxiety that are also common in ASD. Diagnoses are marked with a star (**DIAGNOSIS**). The presence of other interfering distinct anxiety symptoms is indicated by circling the appropriate category.

  - Distinct categories of anxiety include Other Social Fears, Autism-Related Phobias, Focused Interest Fears, Fears of Change, Negative Reactions to Change, and Other Compulsive Behaviors.

## GENERAL ADMINISTRATION NOTES

- Like the ADIS-5-C/P, the ADIS/ASA is a semi-structured interview that allows clinicians to query parents further about their child's behavior after asking a standard set of questions. Guidelines and special considerations are provided at the start of each diagnostic section to help clinicians focus these queries and more effectively differentiate anxiety and ASD features.

- In each section, both required and optional questions are provided in addition to skip-out rules to support an efficient and individualized clinical interview. The interviewer should administer as many optional questions as needed (including at least the first prompt for each question).

- You may administer specific modules of the ADIS/ASA rather than the whole interview, but this may result in an incomplete or inaccurate profile of a child's anxiety. Many children on the autism spectrum who present with one anxiety disorder will meet criteria for another.

## UNDER WHAT CIRCUMSTANCES SHOULD YOU USE THE ADIS/ASA?

### For Whom Is the ADIS/ASA Intended?

The ADIS/ASA is most relevant and useful for children ages 7 to 18 years for whom ASD is suspected or already diagnosed. Additionally, the ADIS/ASA may be clinically useful for youth with more severe intellectual deficits or communication deficits. In general, the interview is useful when careful characterization of the presentation and prevalence of anxiety symptoms in children with more complex developmental profiles is a key concern. For a child without these developmental concerns, the ADIS-5-C/P should be used.

---

**Clinician Note**

*Distinct expressions of anxiety, like those assessed by the ADIS/ASA, may be a more common expression of anxiety in children on the autism spectrum with more severe intellectual disability than disorders like social and generalized anxiety, which can be difficult to assess in nonverbal children. Research on the psychometric properties of the ADIS/ASA and children who are on the autism spectrum and have intellectual disability is ongoing, and expert clinical judgment will need to be exercised to ensure that the developmental level of the child is adequately considered.*

---

## Who Can Administer the ADIS/ASA?

The ADIS/ASA can be administered by professionals with knowledge of and expertise in developmental disabilities, child developmental psychology, and clinical child and adolescent psychology. Trainees with appropriate, expert, and professional clinical supervision who have completed relevant coursework and either clinical or research-level training in the instrument may also use the ADIS/ASA. The usefulness of the ADIS/ASA is contingent on appropriately trained interviewers given the complexity of clinical diagnoses, the interaction of ASD and anxiety, and the semi-structured nature of the interview. This is particularly true for researchers seeking to collect data in a transparent, precise, and structured manner that can be replicated.

## UNIQUE FEATURES OF THE ADIS/ASA

The ADIS/ASA differs from the ADIS-5-C/P standard protocol in the following ways:

- It is specifically designed for assessing anxiety in children on the autism spectrum and contains additional queries and guidelines specific to this group.

- It queries for specific types of anxiety and OCD that are common in children on the autism spectrum rather than the full range of behavioral diagnoses covered in the ADIS-5-C/P. This includes a mix of DSM-5 anxiety disorders and distinct presentation of anxiety specifically indicated for those on the autism spectrum.

- It provides guidance on the differential diagnosis of ASD and anxiety disorders, including methods for evaluating potentially overlapping features (e.g., social avoidance, ruminative thinking).

- It is currently only available as a clinical interview with a parent or primary caregiver and does not include a child interview.

## OVERVIEW OF ADIS/ASA SECTIONS

1. Introduction
2. Developmental and Clinical Concerns and History
3. Academic History and Environment
4. Social Functioning and Other Considerations for Differential Diagnosis
5. Separation Anxiety Disorder
6. Social Anxiety Disorder (Social Phobia) and Other Social Fears
7. Specific Phobias
8. Generalized Anxiety Disorder
9. Fears Related to Focused Interests
10. Fears of Change and Negative Reactions to Change
11. Obsessive-Compulsive Disorder and Other Compulsive Behaviors
12. Additional Other Specified or Unspecified Anxiety Disorders

## DISTINCT ANXIETY AND OTHER SPECIFIED ANXIETY DISORDER

In DSM-5, Anxiety Disorder NOS is replaced by Other Specified Anxiety Disorder; for the latter, clinicians must describe the specific reasons why criteria are not met for any existing anxiety disorder category. Deciding when to use this "Other Specified" category for youth on the autism spectrum is a challenging question given the overlap of anxiety and ASD features and the potential for anxiety to be an integral part of autism. That is, anxiety may be an understandable consequence of the need for sameness or of social deficits, or an expression of general emotion dysregulation inherent to the disorder. In addition to DSM-5 anxiety disorders, many youth on the autism spectrum present with distinct expressions of anxiety that do not meet traditional DSM categories and appear related to or influenced by the cardinal features of ASD (see also Magiati, Ozsivadjian, & Kerns, 2017, for a review). The ADIS/ASA was created to capture these distinct expressions so they can be further studied and addressed clinically. Regardless of their category, these difficulties commonly occur in ASD, are associated with significant distress and impairment, and thus are worthy of assessment.

We recommend that the DSM Other Specified Anxiety Disorder category be reserved for those individuals on the autism spectrum whose distinct fears and worries are:

1. Excessive and overgeneralized, even in light of a child's legitimate social or cognitive differences,
2. More specific than general emotion regulation deficits, and

3. Deserving of targeted, anxiety-based interventions that might not otherwise be implemented.

Accordingly, whether a distinct anxiety symptom, as measured by the ADIS/ASA, translates to a diagnosis of Other Specified Anxiety Disorder should be determined by clinical judgment, weighing the perceived benefits (relative to the costs) of providing a diagnosis for the child in question. For further guidance, see Kerns et al. (2016).

## SCORING INSTRUCTIONS

### General Points

- "Social Functioning and Other Considerations for Differential Diagnosis" (Section 4) is designed to ensure that the clinician understands enough about the child's autism, developmental level, and social experiences to provide an accurate severity rating for specific DSM anxiety disorders and to differentiate anxiety and ASD features as needed.

- Distinct anxiety items (Other Social Fears, Autism-Related Phobias, Focused Interest Fears, Fears of Change and Negative Reactions to Change, Other Compulsive Behaviors, and Other Specified Anxiety) should be reserved for fears, worries, and behavioral manifestations of anxiety that *do not* correspond with traditional diagnostic categories due to their distinct quality or presentation—for example, social fear in a child who does not demonstrate an awareness of social rejection, judgment, or evaluation (see p. 53 in this manual). *These items should not be used for anxiety symptoms that correspond to DSM criteria but lack sufficient severity (CSR < 4) or duration (present for <3 months) to meet full criteria for a diagnosis.* Such symptoms should be given subclinical CSR ratings within their appropriate module.

- *Some but not all other anxiety items are mutually exclusive from the traditional anxiety disorders.* Specifically, a CSR for Other Social Fears should be assigned *only* if the child lacks sufficient social motivation or awareness to qualify for Social Anxiety Disorder. Similarly, Specific Phobias should be designated either within the provided categories or counted as Autism-Related Phobias, not both. By comparison, a child may receive a CSR for *both* GAD *and* Fear of Change or for *both* GAD *and* Focused Interest Fears.

### Overlapping Features and Diagnostic Parsimony

Individuals with anxiety often present with a varied array of worries that may correspond with multiple diagnostic categories. *Efforts should be made to avoid redundancy and double coding of symptoms across diagnoses.* For example, some youth on the autism spectrum may endorse a large number of items in the specific phobias section. Many specific fears may be better conceptualized as a part of GAD if they reflect an overarching, generalized fear of harm to self or others. By comparison, a child with generalized fears about their performance at school and worries about the future with an additional, singular, and severe fear of needles might warrant diagnoses of both GAD and a specific phobia of needles/shots.

*A similar attempt to be parsimonious rather than redundant with diagnoses should be used for the distinct anxiety categories.* Symptoms should be categorized and coded by their overarching motivation and general presentation rather than divided into multiple categories. For example, children who display general fears of novelty and change, including concerns about other *people* because they may change rules, schedules, or expectations, should be coded under Fear of Change. Though these fears include a social element (i.e., the behavior of people), they are most parsimoniously explained by the Fear of Change item. To capture this presentation under Other Social Fears alone would exclude elements of the child's presentation (e.g., general fears of changes in schedule). Further, to code these symptoms in both places would ignore the unifying worry that underlies them—a fear of change that makes both social and non-social endeavors and environments difficult.

## Detailed Scoring Instructions for Specific Items

### *Section 4. Social Functioning and Other Considerations for Differential Diagnosis*

Items in this section are intended to gather information regarding the child's social functioning, sensory sensitivity, and cognitive inflexibility. This will provide an important context for understanding the nature and severity of the child's anxiety and help differentiate difficulties that may be due to ASD from those due to anxiety. For example, understanding the child's interest in social interaction and bullying history will be critical to evaluate the extent to which their social anxiety is not helpful and interfering. Understanding a child's sensory sensitivity and tendency to perseverate will be critical to evaluate the extent to which these difficulties may play into possible Specific Phobias and GAD in later sections. Finally, specific ratings below will also help to capture a distinct presentation of social anxiety in ASD (see the Other Social Fears section), where the child may present as anxious in social situations but is not concerned about negative evaluation or judgment from others and may have limited interest in engaging socially.

### *4.1. Friendships*

This item probes for additional information about the quality and quantity of the child's peer relationships. Clinicians should consider a child's history of successes and struggles to make and maintain friendships when assessing social phobia. Such information will be essential to determining how realistic and proportional a child's social anxiety is given their social experiences and social deficits.

### *4.2. Social Motivation*

This item probes for additional information about the child's base level of social interest and motivation. Assessing social interest and motivation in this explicit way will help the clinician parse out social avoidance due to disinterest (a potential feature of ASD), fears of rejection or ridicule (consistent with Social Anxiety Disorder), or non–evaluation-based social fearfulness and anxious discomfort (consistent with the Other Social Fears category). The child's persistence (or lack thereof) in attempting to initiate social interactions and develop friendships should be taken into account.

## 4.3. Bullying/Peer Rejection

This item probes for additional information about aversive experiences in the child's social history. Clinicians should consider if a child has experienced so significant a bullying history (or ongoing bullying/rejection) that social anxiety is warranted rather than "disordered." To be considered "disordered," social fears should be excessive rather than protective for the child or appropriate given real threats (e.g., excessive bullying). A child with a history of bullying in one situation who now presents with severe social anxiety that has been overgeneralized—resulting in excessive fear of multiple social situations, including nonthreatening ones—should be considered for a diagnosis of Social Anxiety Disorder. By comparison, a child who is being actively bullied at school and worries about attending; who is being mocked, bullied, or laughed at by school peers; and/or who is initially tentative when meeting new peers may not meet criteria for Social Anxiety Disorder due to the realistic and adaptive nature of the fear.

## 4.4. Theory of Mind/Awareness of Social Opinion

This item assesses the child's awareness of social opinions, judgments, and the thoughts of others. Clinicians may use this item to determine whether the child has adequate awareness of the thoughts and feelings of others to meet criteria for conventional Social Anxiety Disorder. Notably, this item is not a measure of empathy. A child may be aware of, but not empathize with, others' thoughts and feelings; likewise, a child may react to the emotions of those around them without being cognitively aware or concerned about those emotions or the thoughts, intentions, and motivations that accompany them. This item pertains specifically to a child's awareness and insight into others' thoughts and feelings about them as an individual. The child's ability to understand *why* individuals have various feelings and thoughts about them or to feel what others are feeling is not necessarily relevant.

## 4.5. Social Opportunity

Clinicians should consider the number of legitimate social opportunities a child has when interpreting their social avoidance and lack of friendships.

## 4.6. Social Scaffolding

A child's social functioning may be potentially overestimated if significant social scaffolding is provided by the parents. This item aims to capture the level of support and structure being provided to ensure that social impairment (due to social anxiety or autism-related difficulties) is not underestimated by the clinician. For example, interference attributable to social anxiety may be underestimated if the parents accommodate the child's anxiety about reaching out to friends by organizing all activities. On the other hand, a child's social motivation (item 4.2) could also be overestimated if the clinician is unaware of the parents' contribution to a child's social success.

## 4.7. General Hypersensitivity

This item inquires into the presence of general as opposed to specific sensory sensitivity—that is, a child who is bothered by most loud sounds, bright lights, scratchy clothes, foods, etc., rather than having an unusual negative response to a specific sound or texture. The item aims to differentiate the presence of general sensory sensitivities from specific phobias of certain stimuli (e.g., specific sounds, sights, or foods). Clinicians *should* code reports of discomfort or irritability to sensations (rather than fearfulness per se) in this item. Children who are both afraid of and generally sensitive to sensory stimuli may be coded here. However, a child who is afraid of loud, unexpected sounds but can easily tolerate loud familiar sounds should *not* be coded on this item. Sensory-seeking behavior may be noted here if introduced by the parent but should not factor into coding.

## 4.8. Perseveration

This item is designed to assess whether the child presents with a generally perseverative or overly focused cognitive style that might contribute to or be mistaken for GAD. Specifically, children who tend to become overly focused on what items or topics are presented to them may appear to be worrying, when, in fact, they are likely to indiscriminately "get stuck" on a positive or negative thought. Similarly, such children may repetitively go over or ask about a past event or upcoming activities not due to worry but due to their general tendency to become fixated. Such behavior may be related to anxiety, intense interests, or the child's efforts to process various information. As such, it is important for clinicians to understand this tendency in a child before assessing the presence and severity of potential worries. A high score on this item would not exclude the diagnosis of GAD—on the contrary, perseverative children may be prone to developing anxiety. Nonetheless, clinicians should be wary of this particular presentation in children on the autism spectrum and its potential to either promote or mimic anxiety difficulties. A key differential may be if the child's perseveration or rumination on a thought causes anxiety and discomfort rather than being somewhat random and circular or even resulting in positive affect.

## Guidelines for the Assessment of DSM-5 and Other Anxiety Symptoms

Guidelines are provided at the beginning of each anxiety disorder and OCD module to aid in the assessment of the diagnosis in children on the autism spectrum. Specific instructions for using these guidelines are also included below.

### Section 5. Separation Anxiety Disorder

Guidelines specific to Separation Anxiety Disorder encourage clinicians to consider (and ask follow-up questions as needed to ascertain) whether the child is legitimately dependent on the parent for any reason, whether the child has reported clear separation worries to the parent or if these worries are simply inferred, and whether there is evidence of clear anticipatory anxiety in the child prior to separation as opposed to only distress in the moment. These questions are designed to aid the clinician in determining whether the child's separation anxiety is excessive given their particular developmental profile and truly consistent with anxiety as opposed to a display of disruptive behavior or generally poor emotion regulation when a routine is changed or the child's expectations are not met.

If Separation Anxiety Disorder criteria are met on the ADIS-5-P, clinicians should consider these guidelines before providing their CSR for Separation Anxiety Disorder. Separation Anxiety Disorder may not be warranted, and an alternate explanation should be considered if the child is legitimately dependent on their parent (e.g., severe communication deficits) or if no clear examples of separation concerns or anticipatory worry about separation can be provided by the parent.

### Section 6. Social Anxiety Disorder (Social Phobia) and Other Social Fears

The Social Functioning section (items 4.1–4.6) should be first completed and referenced when assessing symptoms in this section. Specifically, clinicians should consider if the child's social worries are maladaptive or excessive given their actual social challenges and experiences. In addition, clinicians should be careful to differentiate interference that is related to social anxiety as opposed to difficulties with social communication and engagement characteristic of ASD. Finally, for children who present with anxiety in social situations but do not fear negative evaluation, the Other Social Fears category should be considered in lieu of Social Anxiety Disorder.

The Other Social Fears category allows clinicians to record the severity of social fearfulness that presents in a child with limited baseline social motivation and/or limited awareness of the thoughts, perceptions, and evaluations of others. Fears often center around the child's social confusion—that is, their difficulties reading social cues or knowing what will happen in a social situation.

Clinicians should request a PIR from parents and provide a CSR for Other Social Fears in lieu of Social Anxiety Disorder for children who experience many apparent symptoms of anxiety in social settings (jitteriness, distress, sweating, tension, avoidance) but who do not meet full criteria for Social Anxiety Disorder because they do not show a fear of negative evaluation, embarrassment, or social rejection. Children who score on the Other Social Fears item may appear to be fearful of social situations because of their difficulties navigating such interactions and/or predicting what will happen rather than their concern with or fear of what others may think of them. Similarly, these children may have had very low social motivation from a young age, such that their avoidance of social situations is not clearly due to their concerns about social rejection or ridicule.

Other Social Fears should not be given for children who have limited interest in social situations and therefore frequently avoid or attempt to leave social situations. Rather, Other Social Fears should be reserved for children who not only have limited social motivation but also appear clearly distressed and afraid when in social settings, potentially due to their difficulties anticipating and accurately predicting what will happen or what is expected.

Other Social Fears should be considered in lieu of Social Anxiety Disorder for all children who score at least 2 on the interpersonal relationship items *Social Motivation* and *Theory of Mind/Awareness of Social Opinion*.

Youth on the autism spectrum may report excessive fears about what others may do—for example, such youth may express fears that they may have difficulty navigating a social situation, fears that they may be told off by others, or fears that others will alter or break the rules or expected schedule. Though all these fears may arise in the Social Anxiety Disorder section, they have different motivations and should be differentiated accordingly in the ADIS/ASA.

- Fears of being censured, corrected, or chastised by others often reflect a fear of negative evaluation or negative social performance, consistent with Social Anxiety Disorder. In some cases, the focus of the fear may be around perfectionism, making a mistake, being incorrect, and not meeting the child's personal standard. Such concerns are more consistent with GAD than Social Anxiety Disorder.

- Fears regarding the unpredictability of social situations specifically as opposed to general fears of change or novelty should be coded under Other Social Fears as described above.

- More general worries about rule breaking, unexpected changes, or novelty that include social settings should be coded under the Fear of Change or Negative Reactions to Change items depending on whether or not there is evidence of anticipatory anxiety (see Fear of Change and Negative Reactions to Change sections and notes on "Overlapping Features" above).

### Section 7. Specific Phobias

In addition to the listed specific phobias, clinicians should inquire about and rate phobias that are more common in youth on the autism spectrum, which are listed at the end of the Specific Phobias section in the ADIS/ASA. Examples include fears of beards, mechanical objects, toilets (but attempt to differentiate this from general fear of loud sounds), specific food/textures, cardboard figures, jingles, and specific tones. A child with a general hypersensitivity (item 4.7) to noise with a related fear of loud sounds may receive a typical phobia of loud sounds in the main phobias section. By comparison, a child who is not generally sensitive to sound, but who is terrified of specific songs, tones, or sounds (e.g., a baby crying), should receive a PIR and CSR for Autism-Related Phobia. Interviewers should provide a brief description of the focus of the Autism-Related Phobia within the ADIS/ASA protocol.

### Section 8. Generalized Anxiety Disorder

Items query whether the child has directly reported worries to the parent and whether the child has a legitimate deficit, such as a learning difficulty, that may reasonably contribute to school-based or social concerns. These items are to be reviewed and scored by the clinician prior to the assignment of PIR and CSR ratings for GAD.

Clinicians should assess whether the child has directly or indirectly reported any worries to the parent, or if the worry is entirely inferred by the parent from the child's behavior. If the child has never expressed any worries directly, clinicians should be cautious in assigning a GAD diagnosis.

Children may indirectly report concerns to their parents, for example, by attributing or reporting their fears through a special character (e.g., "Mickey Mouse is afraid"). GAD may be considered if these kinds of reports demonstrate that the child is often worrying, dreading, or anticipating negative events.

GAD should be diagnosed only when a child's fears are excessive and unreasonable, rather than realistic and potentially adaptive. Accordingly, clinicians should query any legitimate struggles the child may be experiencing (e.g., learning difficulties, apraxia, social difficulties, medical issues, physical awkwardness, significant family stress). This knowledge will be essential to determine whether a child's worries are disproportionate given their particular circumstances— for example, children with significant learning or cognitive deficits that influence performance as well as co-occurring anxiety about schoolwork, or children with social deficits who have reasonable concerns about fitting in and future social functioning.

### Sections 9 and 10. Fears Related to Focused Interests, Fear of Change, and Negative Reactions to Change

The ADIS/ASA queries for two distinct anxiety presentations that are often reported by parents of youth on the autism spectrum when inquiring into generalized worry: *Fears Related to Focused Interests* and *Fears of Change*. It also allows the interviewer to evaluate *Negative Reactions to Change* that limit the child's functioning but may not be an expression of anxiety per se.

These items are administered following the GAD section to capture additional fears/ worries or difficulties coping with change that may arise in ASD that are not adequately captured by GAD criteria. Though fears of novelty and change and fears about a focused interest can occur in GAD, along with a variety of others fears, these additional worries or difficulties should receive a unique code for all youth, even those who also meet criteria for GAD. As children with GAD can exhibit these fears with or without co-occurring ASD, the ADIS/ASA assesses each symptom independently so it can be measured and tracked rather than "lost" or subsumed under the GAD category. Whether these presentations deserve a distinct diagnosis, such as Other Specified Anxiety Disorder, when GAD is present, is left to the discretion of the clinician.

*Section 9. Fears Related to Focused Interests*

This section captures excessive worry about losing access or time with a focused interest. If the child presents with generalized anxiety, including fears about their focused interest access or play as well as more traditional worries (e.g., school, future, little things, state of the world), score both the GAD (in the GAD section) and the worry surrounding their focused interest (in this section). If the child presents with excessive worry that is mostly circumscribed to their focused interests, code the symptom only in this section.

*Section 10. Fears of Change and Negative Reactions to Change*

<u>Fears of Change</u>

If there is no evidence of anticipatory anxiety in the child related to change, novelty, or rules, code all parent concerns in the *Reactions to Change* item; however, a child with both anticipatory fears of change and poor reactions to change should be coded here (*Fears of Change* item). Further, perfectionism, a common feature of GAD, should be distinguished from anxiety related to excessive rigidity. Whereas a child with GAD may worry about making things perfect or excelling in all of their endeavors, a child who simply resists change, who adheres to nonfunctional expectations, or who insists that activities be carried out in an exacting manner despite clear imperfection should be coded here.

<u>Negative Reactions to Change</u>

Code this item only if the child has strong reactions to change and is distressed by many of the situations listed in the *Fears of Change* item, but does not worry or express anticipatory anxiety per se. That is, this is a child who has strong reactions (meltdowns, panic attacks) but no significant anticipatory anxiety or avoidance of situations where change might occur. Children with this profile are likely better characterized as having general emotion dysregulation difficulties rather than an anxiety disorder.

If some anticipatory anxiety/worry is apparent, a subclinical code can also be given in *Fears to Change*. However, clinically significant ratings (CSR ≥ 4) cannot be given for both the *Fears of Change* and *Reactions to Change* items. Rather, the *Fears of Change* item should *generally* be used for children who worry about *and* respond with fear and panic to change, and the *Reactions to Change* item should be used for children who have minimal anticipatory worry but significant negative reactions to changes or novelty in their daily life. A child who has significant reactions to rule breaking (but no anticipatory anxiety about rule breaking) and who has anticipatory worries about a different type of change (e.g., changes in daily routine) should be coded under *Fears of Change* solely. Though the anticipation and reactions pertain to different topics, the child should be coded in the *Fears of Change* item because both anticipatory and reactive processes are apparent.

Table 2.1 presents examples of how to determine *Fears of Change* and *Negative Reactions to Change* CSRs.

**TABLE 2.1 Guidelines for Coding Fears of and Negative Reactions to Change**

| Coding Examples | Fears of Change CSR | Reactions to Change CSR |
|---|---|---|
| 1. Child with significant worry about changes in routine and meltdowns in response to changes in routine | ≥4 | 0 |
| 2. Child who consistently becomes anxious and distressed when their schedule is changed, but who does not anticipate or worry about such changes occurring ahead of time | 0 | ≥4 |
| 3. Child who consistently become anxious and distressed when their schedule is changed. Sometimes anticipates or worries transiently about these changes, but worry is minimal and infrequent and does not impair functioning. | 2 | ≥4 |
| 4. Child with excessive worry about changes in routine; frequent checking with parents and teachers to make sure changes will not occur. Child also becomes extremely anxious when rules are broken or changed but does not worry ahead of time about this issue. | ≥4 | 0 |

### Section 11. Obsessive-Compulsive Disorder and Other Compulsive Behaviors

*Obsessive-Compulsive Disorder*

For youth on the autism spectrum, it may be useful to begin with compulsions in the ADIS/ASA section and then inquire into the preceding obsessions. Obsessions may be less apparent or more difficult to assess in this population.

The ADIS/ASA offers the following guidelines for differential diagnosis of ASD and OCD features:

- Obsessions should be clearly distinguished from focused interests. Obsessions reflect unwanted thoughts/images that the child will go to great lengths to alleviate or mitigate as opposed to preferred topics of interest.

- Given that repetitive behaviors are common in ASD and may reflect an intense interest, sensory preoccupation, or self-soothing strategy, repetitive behaviors should not be interpreted as compulsions unless they appear clearly related to "undoing" or "correcting" the obsession in the child's mind.

- Compulsions are different from self-soothing behaviors or repetitive behaviors in that they will be specific to the obsession and triggered by it in addition to having a rigid, potentially ritualistic quality.

Specific probes are provided in the OCD section to help clinicians make these distinctions and differentiate OCD from repetitive/ritualistic behavior in ASD. These probes can be used as needed by the clinician.

*Other Compulsive Behaviors*

If the child presents with ritualistic or compulsive behavior that is associated with distress but falls short of meeting full OCD criteria due to its unusual quality, clinicians may code *Other Compulsive Behaviors*. Clinicians should describe what was distinct about the child's OCD presentation. Examples include verbal rituals (child must recite a specific monologue or complete a specific dialogue with another person in a precise manner and to completion) or compulsive insistence that all doors remain closed or that sleeves be rolled up or down. These compulsive or ritualistic behaviors should be clearly associated with anticipatory distress or discomfort that appears temporarily relieved when the compulsion or ritual is performed but that quickly returns. *This pattern would be coded as* Other Compulsive Behaviors *rather than OCD when the child is unable to articulate or parents are unable to infer why these behaviors are being performed, and particularly if they are related to neutralizing distressing obsessions.* As stated above, repetitive behavior that is associated with positive affect until the child is interrupted (e.g., repetitive lining up of cars that is enjoyable for the child and may result in a tantrum when the child must transition to other activities) should not be coded as OCD.

### Section 12. Additional Other Specified or Unspecified Anxiety Disorders

A section is included at the end of the ADIS/ASA protocol where clinicians can describe and score any additional variants of anxiety that are reported by parents and that do not fit into existing criteria (either traditional or distinct anxiety sections). The current ADIS/ASA distinct anxiety sections reflect symptoms chosen from extensive reviews of the literature, consultation with expert clinicians in anxiety and ASD, and initial research with the ADIS/ASA instrument. Nonetheless, they may not represent a full or exhaustive sampling of the different varieties of anxiety than can manifest in youth. As such, this section allows clinicians to record novel presentations of anxiety in a child and rate their severity (with a unique CSR) so as not to lose information about a child's particular and unusual anxiety presentation. This category also reduces the tendency to add "noise" to existing diagnostic categories by forcing anxiety variants into categories with which they contrast.

## ADDITIONAL READING AND RESOURCES

The following journal article provides further discussion of the ADIS/ASA interview and approach with case illustrations that may be helpful for clinicians:

- Kerns, C. M., Rump, K., Worley, J., Kratz, H., McVey, A., Herrington, J., & Miller, J. (2016). The differential diagnosis of anxiety disorders in cognitively-able youth with autism. *Cognitive and Behavioral Practice, 23*(4), 530–547.

In addition, these articles provide information on the psychometric properties of the ADIS/ASA:

- Kerns, C. M., Kendall, P. C., Berry, L., Souders, M. C., Franklin, M. E., Schultz, R. T., Miller, J., & Herrington, J. (2014). Traditional and atypical presentations of anxiety in youth with autism spectrum disorder. *Journal of Autism and Developmental Disorders, 44*(11), 2851–2861.

- Kerns, C. M., Renno, P., Kendall, P. C., Wood, J. J., & Storch, E. A. (2017). Anxiety Disorders Interview Schedule–Autism Addendum: Reliability and validity in children with autism spectrum disorder. *Journal of Clinical Child & Adolescent Psychology, 46*(1), 88–100.

- Kerns, C. M., Winder-Patel, B., Iosif, A. M., Nordahl, C. W., Heath, B., Solomon, M., & Amaral, D. G. (2020). Clinically significant anxiety in children with autism spectrum disorder and varied intellectual functioning. *Journal of Clinical Child & Adolescent Psychology*, online first: doi.org/10.1080/15374416.2019.1703712